# All My Sizes

*Four Decades of Diet Hell*

Ruth Boehmer, PhD

Copyright © 2012 by Ruth Boehmer, PhD
First Edition – October 2012

Cover illustration by Amber Louie
Author photo by Natalie Santano

**ISBN**
978-1-77097-998-7 (Hardcover)
978-1-77097-997-0 (Paperback)
978-1-77097-999-4 (eBook)

All rights reserved.

This is a non-fiction work. All the people mentioned in the book are real though some have been known to be fake in certain situations. The names used in the book are real names. All the places, meals, and events in this book are real. Any likeness to any other dieting women is not coincidental.

No part of this publication may be reproduced in any form, or by any means, electronic or mechanical, including photocopying, recording, or any information browsing, storage, or retrieval system, without permission in writing from the publisher.

Produced by:

FriesenPress
Suite 300 – 852 Fort Street
Victoria, BC, Canada V8W 1H8

www.friesenpress.com

Distributed to the trade by The Ingram Book Company

# Dedication

To all women everywhere who have ever felt that they were not slim enough, pretty enough, cute enough, smart enough, popular enough, white enough, brown enough, black enough. Welcome to the woman race.

# Introduction

I am an obscure ordinary middle aged woman born and raised in the backest of back woods of British Columbia. I have lived an ordinary working class life, having experienced poverty and prosperity, private school and public school, employment and unemployment, marriage, mothering, divorce, Revenue Canada, and many of the usual vicissitudes of life. I am not a celebrity nor particularly rich or media worthy. I have loved and lost, hated and healed, learned and stumbled upon learning through living the mistakes and missteps of life. Like Eve in her garden, I have eaten much more than my fair share of forbidden food in my own secret gardens.

Through it all I am just an ordinary woman with a very ordinary problem. I suffer from food and weight obsession. I in no way shape or form (pun upon pun piled fatter and deeper), consider myself an expert on diet and weight loss—though experience should certainly provide me with some bit of expertise. I don't even claim to be an expert on MY experience. I am still struggling one day at a time to be at peace with my body and my Maker.

I suppose I have been writing this book for the past forty years, though not intentionally to publish as a book. A veritable record of reality reading, so to speak, much of this book contains my personal journaling about weight and diet issues and the subsequent emotional turmoil of never quite arriving. Like Moses and the children of Israel wandering forty years in the wilderness before finally arriving to the Promised Land, I feel like I have done my time (forty years too!) wandering in the wilderness of weight woes, wondering where that elusive promised land exists—that paradise, free of cellulite, where I can finally arrive, be slim, and have my manna too.

As I have pored over these personal journals from the past in preparation for writing this book, I have noticed several common recurring themes in my life that are boldly and neurotically emblazoned on every page. Using direct journal quotes, I present a four-decade journey of food and diet hell, wrestling over and over again with the same problem. As the years go by, it can be seen that my obsession over weight intensifies as I realize the many repetitive cycles with losing and gaining, becoming despondent at ever conquering the problem. The escalating despair and desperation are almost palpable in many entries as I realize that life is passing ever so quickly and, despite my many diet and exercise programs, I am still fat!

There is no one set mood for the book. Rather, it is a seething pot of multiple moods meshed with numbers on a scale. As the numbers on the scale go down, the mood pendulum swings up; as the numbers on the scale go up, the mood pendulum swings down and out in all directions, cutting a swath of self-loathing, self-destruction, and discord. I have walked (literally) the complete gamut of human emotions, from hilarious laughter to hellish despair and back again, not once, but many times over and over and over again like a neurotic fat rat on a treadmill to hell.

But through it all I can see a common thread, a glimmering glimpse of my indomitable spirit of hope that I will one day (if

I live long enough!) conquer the enemy of my soul. It has been, and continues to be, the worst of times and the best of times.

Several times during this tumultuous journey I have sought a spiritual approach to the problem. Because I am a practising member of The Church of Jesus Christ of Latter-Day Saints (LDS church), I have sought solace and solutions in the familiar faith of my youth. Subsequently, many of my journal entries have morphed into prayers for help in overcoming this habit which has tormented me for the bulk of my life.

For clarification to the reader I explain the regular use of scriptural quotations from the *Book of Mormon* a volume of ancient scripture recording God's dealings with the inhabitants of ancient America, and the *Doctrine and Covenants*, both scriptural books specific to the LDS church. My belief in these scriptures in addition to mainstream Christian scripture—the *Old and New Testaments* has influenced the use of these in my personal pleadings for help in overcoming my food problem. Many of these scriptural quotes have been personalized for me and my weight wilderness.

My maundering on these many scriptures does not, by any stretch of the cellulite, represent official church doctrine and one must not assume that my neurotic sugar-marinated brain interpretations of the scriptures reflect the teachings of the LDS church. They only reflect how these scriptures have spoken to me in my heaviest and lightest of human moments.

The many direct quotes from my journals are by no means representative of my whole life (I actually **did** do other things in my life besides diet and binge, though at times that doesn't seem to be the case). Because this book however, is about my struggle with sizes (many of them), I include only the many journal entries dealing with my weight obsession. Some descriptions of life situations are necessarily included to set the context of my food benders, including the ups and downs of my weight.

Simply looking around me in my community and the larger world of media, I can see clearly that I am not unique in these weight struggles. Therefore I hope that my writings will resonate with other women who have spent decades of their lives struggling with their weight, ever dieting, but never quite able to come to that promised land of eternal slender.

It is also my hope that younger women struggling with weight issues will read and see the futility of dieting and the many empty promises perpetuated by the diet industry. I hope that they will read about my journey and look deep within their souls to find out what is really at the core of their food and weight issues. Perhaps this book will influence them to not start that first diet, subsequently triggering a cascade of diet hell which can plague them for decades. To them I say, please look deep within your soul and see your beauty and the power of balance and positive health habits in caring for your precious body. Learn and develop healthy ways to cope with the challenges of life and love yourself through the journey. Above all, surround yourself with the love of God evidenced in loving people who feed your eternal soul. Do not spend your money and strength on that which has no worth (crazy diets), nor your time with people who suck the God-given light right out of your soul.

This book is naturally disorganized to represent the insanity and turmoil of dieting and binging. It is reality reading. There are no chapters so to speak, only journal entries along with descriptions and reflections necessary to set the context of the coincident diet or binge. I guess it then becomes a biography of sorts, or rather, dietography; or foodography; or weightography, if I may butcher the English language to suit my needs.

I am ashamed that so much of my life energy went into battling and tormenting myself over my weight; it was such a waste of joy and peace. Some journal entries expose the volatile neuroticism of my obsession, while other entries are admittedly senseless drivel. I am tempted to remove these entries; however the authenticity of the journey would be greatly threatened. I am what I am. I wrote what I felt. I wrote what I thought. I wrote what I prayed. All of this was written in the moment that I felt and thought and prayed it. From adolescence to middle age, it is all spelled out there in black and white, spanning the depth and breadth of human emotion, a veritable open wound begging to be healed.

Read to learn; go forth to live.

# Fat before I came forth from my mother's womb

They said I was well over nine pounds at birth—not **under** ten pounds, but well **over** nine pounds. There's something so ominous about using the word 'over' rather than the word 'under'. I'm not sure why that is.

So I could say that I started out overweight—more than expected and wired for growing. My mom didn't breast feed me for whatever reasons, known more to her than anyone else. I could excuse my weight problems by blaming it on her, but the fact is she didn't breast feed any of her nine children (I am number four)—most of whom have not struggled with weight issues. But **I'm** not bitter! Perplexed, but definitely NOT bitter.

Bitter or not, I have questions about the environment of that womb that nurtured me. Why I ask, did I get so big in there? My mom was a small woman. My family lived a rather subsistence-type lifestyle, living off the family cow, chickens, and garden. Where did all that fat come from before I was even born? Was I grabbing food that belonged to my mom, making her a rake while I sucked the life out of her? If only I had kept a journal of those nine months I might know. However, I am left only to my speculative imagination.

Was I simply an easy keeper from conception? What can I say? How could I take responsibility for my birth weight? Was I a glutton before I was born? Did I suck the fat right out of my mom's cells from conception to birth?

Was I born with this weakness? According to *Book of Mormon* doctrine, my weaknesses are God given (Ether 12:27), not that that is an excuse to never conquer them, but it does give me food for thought as to my size at birth. Who was I before I was born and how did this become my weakness? Obviously, these are questions that I cannot answer for now and I really don't have any recall of my intrauterine life. If I did I would have written a book a long time ago—*My Nine Months of Binging In Utero*, or *Diary of a Fat Fetus*.

# Leaving the womb but not the fat

After nine months of uterine bliss freeloading off my mom, I came out one sunny Sunday afternoon in the fall of 1955—"well over nine pounds" they said, and ready to eat.

My mom doesn't share many memories of that day, except that she says she looked out the window of her bedroom (I was born at home) just after my birth and saw a man she loathed (not my dad!) walking up the sidewalk—such a pleasant memory. It was like the black raven of fat hell was hovering over my birthday, the very demon of fat waiting to pounce and plump up my fat cells.

My first food source was the family cow—raw milk from my very first meal. By all accounts I should be dead rather than struggling with weight all my life. However, I not only lived, but thrived too well on the rich Jersey cow milk abundant on the farm. My one picture as a baby about nine months old shows a rolly polly bald Buddha look-alike, sort of like the Jersey calves that shared their mother's milk with me. They had four stomach chambers to digest their milk and I had only one. Maybe that's why I look like I have four chambers in my middle—nature evolved them for me to deal with the cow's milk. It could also have something to do with my propensity to eat with the herd.

Early childhood pictures, though rather scarce, do reveal a consistently chunky girl. Though I did not give my size a tremendous amount of thought then, I was aware of comments made by visiting relatives who affectionately labelled each of my mom's nine children to keep the brood straight. They referred to me as the husky one, the easy keeper, the plump one and, more pointed, the fat one with freckles.

I don't recall resenting these comments, but they certainly cemented my belief that I was the husky one. Their comments simply made me aware that relatives noticed my size in comparison to siblings. One portly aunt, when visiting and listening to such comments, defended me saying:

"We're not fat, we're just muscular with big bones."

I still recall exactly where I was sitting in the house when she said that. It was one of those profoundly pivotal moments in life, like when JFK was assassinated. It might have been that same year too. For some reason her comment gave me a sense that something about my size had to be defended. Alarmed, I wondered what it was about me that was defective and needed to be defended. In retrospect I can feel for my portly aunt who had likely had years of struggling with her weight and strongly empathized with my fat plight.

# Fat sheep of the family

I had some thin sisters who were referred to as the pretty ones, so I got the message early in life that the husky one was not the pretty one. I recognized early that I ate faster than my thin sisters. On rare occasions when we had cheese (more JFK moments), which was like gold to us, we were each rationed a portion to eat. I gulped mine down so fast that I barely tasted it, while my older thin sister ate hers slowly, savouring every bite. When my cheese was gone, I watched in agony while she calmly enjoyed her share, tormenting me with every bite. I always puzzled that she could eat such a treat so slowly. It was sheer agony for my cheese-craving soul.

My childhood diet leaned heavily on starchy foods. Potato soup thickened with fresh cream was a staple and quite often what we ate every day along with heavy homemade brown bread and home churned butter. For years it seemed to be my chore to spread the slices of bread with butter before they were put on the table. I had a habit of taking a bite out of each slice as I spread it with butter. Despite my grandmother's scolding me with each bite I took, I seemed not to be able to butter a single slice without taking a bite out of it. I was frequently full before the meal began, then sat and ate with my family, habitually the last one to leave the table.

Dessert was usually home canned fruit smothered in heavy fresh cream. Best dessert ever! I wish I had some now. There never seemed to be a scarcity of it. My family lived simply yet richly where cream, butter, and bread were concerned. It was a simple life, yet rather fattening—at least for me, the husky one.

Strangely the one food from my childhood that I absolutely hated, oatmeal porridge, is the one food that has since been extolled, exalted, and damn near enshrined as the ultimate health food for the heart and hips and bowels and brain—and pancreas and liver and fingers and toes and eyelashes too. Who'd have thought? I hardly dare to admit publicly and in writing that I hated rolled oat porridge. The only way my mom got me to eat it was by smothering it in brown sugar and that rich Jersey cream. Even then I used to gag over it and vowed every day that one day when I had the choice I would never eat oatmeal porridge again. Like many of my impulsive vows, I have since eaten (literally) these words as well.

Vows or no vows, I knew I was different where food was concerned. It seemed to have a stronger hold over me than it did my sisters close in age. I knew that I ate more than they did and it never seemed to be an issue except when pointed out by visiting relatives. The more it was pointed out, the more I ate. Sometimes I resorted to eating where no one would see. This involved sneaking food from the kitchen and taking it to my bedroom to hide and eat. It was my own personal version of hide and sneak.

Fortunately candy was scarce in our family. Except for Christmastime, I don't recall having an abundance of candy or pop or juice of any sort. When Christmas candy was available I ate it with great gusto and always seemed to get a 'sour' stomach, belching what tasted and smelled like rotten egg smell. I'm not sure what this meant, but I believe that I had trouble with sugar then and have certainly continued with such through most of my life.

## Memories light the corner of my thighs

There was a time when I was around eleven that I spent a week away from home visiting with a cousin. It was the longest, most homesick week of my childhood. I have two prominent memories from that week. Both incidentally have to do somehow with food and fat. One was when my cousin and I went to the public pool to swim. Two boys were taunting her and calling her fat. She was fatter than me (probably had something to do with why I liked her). I screamed at the boys who seemed bent on tormenting her. This just set me up to be included as a victim of their bullying. I don't mean to be vindictive, but I hope they're fat now.

My other memory of that experience was the awful spell that white bread held over me. I had never before seen or eaten store-bought white bread and I couldn't seem to get enough of it. I was sneaking that bread every chance I got and I couldn't seem to ever feel like I had enough to eat. I'm sure my aunt fed me, but I seemed to want to eat all the time and it was that white bread that I kept sneaking out of the cupboard and stuffing in my face.

I felt ashamed and guilty for sneaking it and hiding in the bathroom to eat it but I could not seem to stop the compulsion. Maybe it was emotional eating because I was terribly homesick and felt like I was away from home forever instead of just one week. It seemed that food was my security. But more than that, that white bread triggered a biological craving inside of me for more and more and more, without ever being satisfied. Broccoli never did that to me, neither then or now.

It seems that some form of food addiction was evident in my childhood. If so, adolescent dieting set the stage for replacing a food addiction with a diet addiction.

# Ruth, plain and fat.

As I got into my teens I became more aware of my size in comparison to others. I was a husky girl, no doubt about it. A husky girl with thin sisters and that seemed to accentuate my bulky size. For my childhood years, that seemed okay. I could beat the boys in arm wrestles, climb trees with the best of them, ride horses, cows, bulls, sheep—whatever. I was happy in my husky self and I didn't seem to care that I was a plain, husky, strong girl.

Enter hormones, that curse of the endocrine system and thief of childhood fantasy. Suddenly I wasn't just a husky girl, I was a husky pubescent girl with breasts and hips and hair where I had never seen it before. It wasn't enough just to beat the boys at arm wrestles anymore. Now I wanted to be something different. I wanted to be a girl! All of this seemed to accentuate the fact that I was fat.

Though not recorded in any journal, I do recall my first attempt to reduce food to lose weight sometime in my fifteenth year. All I recall is that I starved myself briefly in hopes of being skinny, but quickly abandoned the attempt. I knew it wouldn't last and I could never really be anorexic (something I had never heard of at that point).

During these years I was taking piano lessons from a delightfully plump woman. Despite seeming to be constantly on a diet, she remained the same plump size during the four-plus years she was my piano teacher. I doubled as her babysitter and was fascinated with her diet candy AYDS. While babysitting I would sneak those tasty chocolate candies in the hopes that they would make me magically and permanently slim. They didn't. Neither she nor I got slim eating those infernal candies, but I did learn to play the piano beautifully. For that I will always hold my piano teacher, fat or thin, dear to my heart.

In the summer I was fifteen my life took a decidedly different turn when I left the insulated polygamous community of my birth and went out into the big wide world of the town people (Creston—population 3000), starting public school in my grade eleven high school year. In a personal sense it was akin to leaving the womb again.

# Leaving the womb again
# (still well over nine pounds!)

Outside the cocoon of familiarity I struggled to find my secure place in life. I had few social skills, fewer fashion skills, and was awkward as hell. I struggled to fit in socially as much as I did to fit into my clothes, which were decidedly different from the outside world. When I left the community and started wearing pants, I felt very self-conscious, like my butt was extremely conspicuous. My butt and arms seemed to be my main concern as I always seemed to have large, and what I perceived to be, hairy arms.

Probably no one even gave my arms a second glance, but I sat in class feeling painfully conspicuous and out of place. I couldn't wait to get home at the end of each day to the comfort and acceptance of fresh bread and honey. There's nothing like the aroma of grandma's whole wheat bread baking in the oven and the first slice smothered in homemade butter and honey. It was bread and honey for the soul after a day of feeling taunted, alone, and ugly at school.

My first written recorded hint of angst over my body size is recorded in a letter I wrote to my older sister when I was fifteen. She had married and moved away the previous year. Her leaving had left a huge hole in my heart (but not my belly or thighs) and may have contributed to my attempt to fill that hole with food. This letter was written shortly after I started public school, and I STILL love ice-cream.

<u>September 20, 1971</u>

I don't know what I did today that was interesting, fun, and exciting, but I did buy me a 20¢ tiger ice cream cone and I'm getting fatter too.

I'm not sure why I would feel the need to tell my sister that I was getting fatter—perhaps because she was the thin one and the teen confidante that I shared my deepest and innermost angst with.

Along with her, my weight is also mentioned in an old school paper that I had written for a grade eleven English class on what I would do if I had only two months to live. It doesn't surprise me that food was front and center in my dying plans. I have no idea why this paper was kept all these years, but it was. Perhaps I held on to obscure things like I held onto my fat.

<u>November 1, 1971</u>

What would I do if I had only two months left to live? To tell you the truth, I don't know what I would do because no person can really predict what he will do under certain circumstances. However, I will predict as accurately as possible what I would do knowing I had only two months to live.

First, I would go with my family to Hurricane, Utah, where we could be with my sister and her husband's family. While down there I would continue my church and school activities the best I could. I would write a diary of my life. I'd try to keep an attitude that death is really quite painless and maybe I'd be better off dead.

> I'd eat all sorts of good things such as bananas and grapes, and I wouldn't even watch my weight, except to see it go way up. On the last day, I'd repent and ask forgiveness of God for any wrongs I ever did. I'd die playing the piano.

I'm not sure why bananas and grapes were the two good things I included in my deathbed diet, but probably because we rarely could afford such food luxuries when I was that age. Even now I would think dying at my piano surrounded by grapes and bananas would be a most pleasant way to go.

Just a few months later, another letter to the same sister records reference to my size.

> <u>January 15, 1972</u>
>
> Oh stink: I just popped my pants again. I think I better lose some weight before I have to redo my wardrobe.

Those pants were likely the only cool pants I had to wear to school, and as I recall they were some of those coveted bell bottom jeans. My sister had given them to me so that I could blend in with the public school kids and avoid some of the taunting and rejection I felt in my first year of public school. Those jeans were flipping sacred and I couldn't grow out of them—likely why they were the topic for discussion in my letter. Something about poverty helps a person remember exactly what pants she had (note to self, poverty rocks). I can say that now, but as a teenager it was very difficult to feel awkward, fat, unattractive, and poorly dressed.

# That which doesn't kill me makes me eat.

The most painful was taunting from teenage boys. I had a crush on one guy for my two years of public high school. Not surprisingly, he never paid any attention to me, never even a nod my way, despite having several classes together and a common passion for music. Not that I'm bitter or anything, but he dated a skinny girl. I wasted two years of my precious youth pining for him, certain that if I were slim he would want me.

One of my most painful feel-ugly days was during grade eleven when I was wearing those bell bottom pants my sister had given me and I finally felt cool. As I followed a group of popular girls in the school hallway, a group of boys (including the one who held my heart hostage for two years) were standing sentinel, commenting on each girl that walked by. For each of the girls in front of me, they whistled and shouted, "How sweet it is". When I walked by, one voice cruelly shouted, "How sweet it isn't", punctuated with group laughter. It was a humiliating and emotionally devastating day in my life, further reinforcing my self-belief that I was fat and ugly. I regret I even gave those guys a second thought, let alone allowed their cruelty to define me. But sixteen year old girls' hearts and minds are very tender and vulnerable to the opinions of others, especially guys. Sad but true.

Following this heart wrenching humiliation, I once again decided to try my luck at losing weight, deciding to go one week eating only food I could drink. A friend had bet me that I couldn't do it, so I swore on a stack of bread and cheese (metaphorically speaking) that I could. I didn't make the full week and caved at five days, starving and stupidly thinking I was going to solve my weight problems once and for all. Needless to say, it didn't. What it did do was awaken the feeding monster living inside my psyche and ignited a flame of food obsession.

# Ass of 73

But even with all that, look at this journal entry from the summer of 1973, the year I graduated from Prince Charles Secondary School. I weighed 130 pounds! At 5'4" I wouldn't really be considered fat at this weight. Yet I remember feeling so fat and ugly. I would see myself as an absolute rail now if that is what I weighed.

This journal entry refers to a trip to Vancouver, British Columbia, when I was required to have a complete physical assessment prior to being accepted into the Vancouver General Hospital (VGH) School of Nursing.

August 28, 1973

Weight 130 pounds—60 kg.

My best friends in high school were much thinner and smaller than I. They never seemed to obsess about food, and I marvelled at that. I remember one time they were at my house for dinner. Immediately after a huge Thanksgiving dinner I picked up an apple and started to eat. My dear thin friend innocently asked me, "How can you be hungry and eat that apple after such a big meal?" Something about that question just stunned me and I thought—what does hunger have to do with anything? It seemed rather revelatory that hunger would be the motive for eating an apple. I just wanted to eat it, and that's what I did.

I managed to eat my way through high school surrounded by loving family, a few good friends, and a new church community. My mother and my faith in God introduced me to the mainstream LDS church, which I joined in the summer of 1973. Filling my faith void, I continued to write my desires for perfection.

I seemed to be very much an idealist, eschewing realism, ever looking for the perfect self. As a goal-oriented person I sincerely wanted to improve myself. Perhaps my methods were not always effective nor was my weak flesh always accommodating to such grandiose ideals. Still, my spirit was strong and my desire to be a disciplined ideal person persisted.

In the months following my high school graduation I worked at a local hardware store while waiting to start nursing school in February 1974 at VGH. My journal entry on New Year's Day 1974 shows a typical hope-filled plan for my future. It is also typical of the all-or-nothing mentality that has plagued much of my life.

January 1, 1974

> Another year is ahead of me and I am confident that I will progress in it. Bettering myself is a chief goal. This year it is my resolution to eat no chocolate or anything that contains cocoa. A body has to be fit to live with God. I am what I eat, and I want to be good.

All the hope and goal writing in the world could not have prepared me for the emotional challenges ahead.

# Way out of the womb

In February of 1974, at age eighteen, I moved to nursing residence in Vancouver, British Columbia (a ten hour drive from my home town). Not only was I leaving the security of my small community and relocating to a large city, I was also taking on training for a career that I knew very little about. In short, I hadn't a clue what I was getting into and how it would challenge my mental, spiritual, and physical health. As usual I had high hopes of finding the fountain of fitness and getting thin while away at school.

What I found was a whole new way of eating and a bounty of food like I had never seen before. With an unlimited cafeteria ticket and a host of foods available, I quickly began packing on the pounds. The dorm kitchens were stocked with bread, peanut butter, and jams. While other girls went out partying on weekends, I ate and studied, and ate and studied, and ate and studied some more. Toast with peanut butter and red currant jam filled my lonely nights far from home. I recall eating whole loaves of bread, frequently emptying the kitchen.

During the five months I spent in nursing school in Vancouver I have two records of dieting hopes: one a journal entry and the other a letter to my sister.

<u>March 14, 1974</u>

I'm glad that I am on a diet to lose weight so I can really get in shape. I'm glad that I can take karate lessons for free here in residence.

I have absolutely no recall of those karate lessons, which is likely why I never lost weight.

<u>March 15, 1974 [letter to my sister]</u>

On Wednesday I went to see the head nurse in residence and got a diet from her. Its a thousand calories a day diet and I'm to weigh once a week and report my weight. I sure hope I lose weight finally. Also, I'm walking up the stairs instead of taking the elevator. After walking up six flights of stairs, I'm almost dead with fatigue.

There is no more mention of my dieting days in Vancouver, however I do remember that when I went home at Easter I was considerably heavier than when I had left home in February. My memories of the months in Vancouver are decidedly dark and dreary – somewhat like the weather.

In June of that year my father died of leukemia. I was plagued with homesickness and fear and loneliness, finally ending in a withdrawal from the nursing program. Not only did I not succeed at dieting, I did not succeed at nursing either. I posted a final note on my dorm door—gone with the wind to the prairie provinces.

# Diets blowing in the wind

Following withdrawal from the nursing program in Vancouver I went directly to Lethbridge, Alberta (a five hour drive from home) to attend college there. Fortunately I was able to get in to the nursing program and stay with some friends (the thin friends) who had moved there after graduation. Filled with hope once again, I set out on a new venture hoping that this would magically transform the person I was and did not want to be into that idealistic perfect (read, *slim*) person.

Once again my January journal entry records hope for getting slim once and for all. This seemed to be most unpleasant as I white-knuckled my way through the food deprivation process, succeeding only for short periods of time. At the time I lived with friends who were perennially thin and never seemed to have any issues with food or weight (damn them!), something that is a total enigma for me. I was always torturing myself and suffering over food—too much or too little but never quite just right. In addition to food restrictions, I did try to engage in regular exercise as evidenced by my journal entries.

January 13, 1975

I'm on a diet. I want to weigh 120 pounds by next summer so I've been eating less—no sugar or honey. I always leave the table hungry, but I just try to keep in mind an image of being skinny—well, slim anyway.

April 1, 1975

I made supper tonight then did some exercises. It took all my strength to refrain from eating before supper but I did it. I want so bad to lose some weight, but when the old stomach gets contracting and growling, I almost die—well, not that bad.

April 4, 1975

My skinny friend got me up early to go jogging and was it ever cold, snow blowing in our faces, but we did it and felt great.

April 17, 1975

I jogged around the trailer court today. I still feel a bit sacked out from it and from the fifty jumping jacks I just did.

Once again my dieting efforts failed or I failed at them. Either way the results were the same—I was actually fatter after the diet than before it. In the spring of 1975 I was doing a nursing practicum in the Claresholm Care Center in Claresholm, Alberta. While there practising in a unit for seniors with dementia, I was one day grabbed by a little old lady who pulled me onto her lap. While squeezing my hips she said, "You're what we call in the cattle industry an easy keeper," (I DID say she was demented right?). I was mortified! My size was once again brought to the forefront and by summer time I was once again desperate to be thin, as recorded in this journal entry.

June 21, 1975

I hate it when I feel fat. I just feel so ugly and sloppy. I've just got to lose weight this summer.

This was my only entry about weight for the rest of that year. The summer passed with little change to my size and I returned to college in Lethbridge in the fall.

## Definitely NOT a dress size

While back at college, I desperately wanted to go to a special church dance but did not have an appropriate dress (the part of poverty that doesn't rock). A friend and fellow student in nursing allowed me to borrow a beautiful red velvet dress she had. Off I went to the dance, knowing that I was too fat for that dress and that I was bursting its seams. During the dance, my underarm perspiration leaked the color of the red velvet into the white of the sleeves and my bulk tore the fabric underarm seams. I was mortified, ashamed, fat, and generally hideous for insisting on wearing a dress that was clearly too small. I offered to pay for the dress, which was basically irreparable with the damage I had caused. The friendship ended. I ate. I felt humiliated and full of self-loathing for trying to fit into something I knew was too small but that I desperately wanted to wear. I lost a good friend (wish I had lost weight instead).

Shortly thereafter, I was once again planning a thousand calorie diet, this time joining with other family members. So what did I **not** learn from the previous diets that had failed?

> February 28, 1976
>
> Mom, my sister, and I decided that we would go on a thousand calorie diet to get down to our optimum weights, and then we'll all get a new spring dress.

It seems that at some point of failure at losing weight I simply decided to start dressing differently, as indicated in this next entry. Perhaps a change in fashion would make me look the thin part I yearned to be. If I couldn't change my size, I would change my manner of dressing. Certainly that would make all the difference. I could have my cake and wear it too.

March 8, 1976

I think I'll start wearing dresses to school. They make me look slimmer.

Not long after this entry I have recorded some deeper insightful thoughts about my eating problem. I seemed to bounce between one extreme and another, never quite finding a sensible balance or healthy relationship with food. Even at age twenty I realized the harmful emotional and spiritual effects of excess food, yet still seem plagued with its powerful pull.

April 3, 1976

I have a problem controlling my appetite and often find myself overeating to the point of sickness. I know I must conquer this for I do not feel close to God when I am in such a state, so here it goes. First, I will not pick into dough or any food while I am preparing it—that's a terrible fault I have—always eating while I make stuff e.g. like bread or cookies etc. Second, I will exclude, banish, and exterminate chocolate from my diet at all costs. Chocolate is out!

Such an entry is so typical of my all-or-nothing approach to living life and of the futility of my many written goals for changing. I was much better at writing goals and plans than I was at following and reaching them, at least weight loss goals that is. Though I never managed to graduate from fat hell that year, I did manage to graduate from college with a diploma in nursing, launching me into the next era of dieting.

# Ass of 76

Between the last entry and the next I graduated from college as a registered nurse. While searching for a dress uniform to wear for the ceremony, my number one concern was, you guessed it, how to look thinner than I was. At the suggestion of my presumed wiser, skinnier roommate, I purchased a pattern and fabric she assured me would be slimming. I hated the pattern and the fabric, but the people pleaser in me would not let me say it out loud so I went along with my roommate to keep the peace.

When I had finished sewing the uniform, I tried it on and felt horribly fat in it, so I went out and bought one at the uniform shop. I still felt fat at my graduation. That's about my most prevalent memory of the occasion—I felt fat. That and the director of nursing mispronounced my name and announced that I was from Alberta. I don't mean to be rude, but please! Fat or thin, a girl raised in the majestic mountains of beautiful British Columbia does NOT want to be mistaken for a prairie girl.

Though I have no record of my actual weight then, I recall it being around 150 pounds, a weight I find quite palatable now, but certainly not the 130 pounds I was at my high school graduation. In the three years from high school grad to college grad, I had managed to diet myself up by twenty pounds. Things were getting bad. Now I really was overweight!

After graduation I returned to the security of my home and started my nursing career in the Creston hospital. To coincide with my launch into nursing, I launched on yet another plan to lose weight.

This time I was quite successful to the point of getting into my younger sister's pants. It was a heady experience and I remember distinctly vowing that, as God is my witness, I will never be fat again! It felt so good to be thin that I couldn't imagine ever allowing myself to gain weight again. Ah, if only. It's a blessing at times that we are not given a glimpse of the future. Had I known that I had more than thirty years of diet hell ahead of me, I may have just eaten myself into oblivion, slit my throat, and gone out in a binge of glory.

Several months passed without record of my weight woes. The year ended with a brief summary of the summer of 1976, the year I started my career as a registered nurse.

<u>December 31, 1976</u>

Summer memories of Arrow Creek swimming, dairy queening with my thin friend and trying to lose weight. Lost a few pounds.

Despite my vow that I would never be fat again, the slim thing did not last as I had anticipated. Less than a year went by before I recorded another goal to lose weight. I have probably been on at least one thousand, thousand calorie diets!

<u>September 19, 1977</u>

Today my goals are to lose fourteen pounds by Christmas. My thousand calorie diet begins today and

I will not allow myself to splurge until Thanksgiving and that is my only splurge day.

Between that diet and the next I moved to Nanaimo, British Columbia, for a nursing job there. It is still a mystery to me why I ever made this move to the west coast, alone and away from family and friends again. My younger sister and I lived together in an apartment in the rain drenched city, wondering with each passing day what the hell we were doing there besides eating.

December 10, 1977

My sister and I both started a thousand calorie diet today.

The stay in Nanaimo was short lived (like my diets), and within a short while I had a target date and target weight for returning home. Once again I wanted desperately to return home a thin person. The next few journal entries focus on this desire and again the struggles with diet hell.

December 22, 1977

Today I'm disgusted with myself for over-eating. There are all kinds of goodies at work, which I indulged in, then ate more when I got home. I'm for sure starting an eight hundred calorie diet right this moment. I've simply got to lose ten pounds before I go home the end of January.

December 24, 1977

Today I am so happy for resisting all the treats at work. I just kept thinking ahead to being slim. I would much rather have the joy of being slim than eating 'til I'm sick. I'm on an eight hundred calorie diet until the end of January. By then I hope to weigh 128 pounds and will increase to a thousand calories until I weigh 120 pounds, then go on a levelling number of calories.

As previously mentioned, I had wonderful grandiose plans written and details of how I would accomplish my goals but something was just missing (common sense, anyone?).

While in Nanaimo, my sister and I were invited to an elderly church member's place for Christmas dinner. Her kindness and generosity proved the downfall of yet another best laid plan for dieting.

December 25, 1977

I really pigged out. Our fellow church member had gone to so much work preparing supper that I thought it would be selfish to refuse. After all her kindness I would hate to hurt her.

The people pleaser in me comes out in that entry—not that the food didn't influence my easy to be entreated submissiveness.

Once Christmas was over, it was back to dieting as usual.

December 29, 1977

I've stuck to my reducing diet for four days now. My reward for going a week and a half is a perm. I can't reward myself with food, so I'll do it with pride and self-respect. It all helps to improve my morale.

After leaving Nanaimo in early 1978 I set off for Utah to seek other adventures where my older sister lived. Still after that elusive diet to end all diets, my struggles with food continued. The next few journal entries were written while visiting with a family of a missionary I had known in Creston.

February 24, 1978 Kaysville Utah

I'm thoroughly disgusted with myself for pigging out. I really hate myself when I lose control of my appetite.

February 25, 1978

My sister and I went shopping with an acquaintance —had a great time. We went through a delicatessen shop and sampled all their goodies. In a t-shirt and jeans shop my friend pointed out the words to me, "We alter bottoms". As we laughed at this, I said, "Let's go have ten pounds taken off ours." More laughing and jokes continued.

Sure I could laugh on the outside, but inwardly I was already weary with weight woes and weeping inconsolably. My travels continued as I searched for the right place for me to land and be me.

The following journal entries were written while travelling alone by car.

March 27, 1978

I travelled to Ricks College, ten hours – a very uneventful trip. I over-ate all the way.

March 28, 1978

I travelled on to Kaysville, Utah, but this time I kept on a diet. I nibbled on cauliflower instead of taco chips— felt good for doing it.

As a 22 year old single LDS female I was beginning to feel the pressure of being single, further reinforcing my feelings of being undesirable and alone. The need to be thin intensified as I aged (okay, I was only 22, but 22 and single in LDS society is just **not** cool). I was facing that which I feared most coming upon me – being an old maid (okay, that and being fat!).

## I'm a little bit genetic; I'm a whole lot psyche and soul.

Besides a dieting fixation, I had a find-a-husband fixation too. This included a fixation with the Osmond's, especially Jay. I thought that if I could just be slim enough and pretty enough then serendipitously run into him, he would fall madly in love with me and I would live happily married and slim ever after.

All my problems would magically disappear and I would be that elusive person I struggled to find somewhere there buried in all my emotional identity baggage. This journal entry records my Osmond plan. I have even set a specific time limit for this goal and still I failed to reach it. Screw the experts!

March 30, 1978

By mid-June I will be beautiful slim, have a nice trim hair style, and be a cosmetics expert. Then I shall meet Jay.

Foolishly I disclosed this dream to a male acquaintance who commented, "You're not bad, but a little porky for him". Such a hurtful comment inevitably sent me plummeting into a vat of something delicious to eat, which ended up once again into the abyss of food hell—food never said such hurtful things to me and it didn't care if I was single or married.

At this point in my life, I started working as a nurse at Utah Valley Hospital in Provo, Utah, hoping to find that elusive perfect Mormon man (aka, Jay Osmond) to marry. I lived there briefly in a dorm shared with other single women. My social life revolved around church functions in Provo. My journaling for this period indicates a desire to be of optimum beauty and health, filled with hope again for that elusive beauty I wanted to be. Ever dreaming but never quite making the dream.

April 1, 1978

At a social event a few times I was tempted to indulge in the sweet refreshments, but my thought quickly turned to higher sites. I want to marry a beautiful body, so I'm going to be a beautiful body.

April 4, 1978

This evening I began a special exercise program. I got the book *Cellulite* and am following its exercises.

April 5, 1978

A couple little boys came to the door selling candy for some boys' organization. I couldn't say no, so I bought a box for $2.00. I didn't eat a one, but put them out for my roommates.

Somewhere in the four days between that entry and this one, something occurred to bring on the food again. I was probably just tired of depriving and starving myself. Even with that relapse, I always had the hope and optimism that I would conquer.

## April 9, 1978

I am tired and disgusted that I blew my diet, but I'm reminded of a Richard L. Evans quote, "Just because you may have taken one step down the wrong road does not mean you have to take two."

# Have binge will travel

Somewhere between April and June I moved on to Hurricane, Utah, where my sister lived and got a nursing job at Dixie Medical Center in St. George. My diets and failures were about as unpredictable as my moves from place to place. Perhaps looking for that place that would make me what I thought I wanted to be. With each new move came new hope that this would be the catalyst for freeing the beautiful butterfly hidden beneath the insecurities of the past and the cocoon of cellulite. Always optimistic that something would magically happen to get that fat off for good, I continued to set lofty goals for myself.

June 22, 1978

I have been lying in bed meditating on reforms I must make in my life. Refrain from overindulging in food. Regularly exercise body physically.

June 26, 1978

Today I feel great. I started tennis lessons. I felt a bit awkward there, but hope to improve. I also joined the health spa—wow, what a great, great feeling. I exercised for about 1 ½ hours then went into the steam room and whirlpool. I felt so clean and invigorated. It makes me realize how important physical well-being is to spiritual and emotional well-being. I'm so excited to be on an exercise and diet program—this time it's for good. I will not harm my body with junk food and laziness.

It's interesting to observe my habits—i.e. when I don't control my appetite for food I lose self-control and respect in other areas.

My goal is this: to weigh 115 pounds by my 23rd birthday. That gives me exactly fifteen weeks and I know I can do it.

115 pounds! I don't think I have weighed that little since I was ten. What was I thinking? No wonder I had such trouble ever achieving my goals. They were just plain ridiculous for the most part. But I dieted on, always certain that I was going to be that waif I thought I needed and wanted to be. I would work a night shift then head for the gym to work out as recorded in this next entry.

June 29, 1978

This morning I am sitting in the St. George city park waiting until the health spa opens at 9:00 a.m. I got off work at 7:15 a.m. then practised tennis for a while, but it wasn't much fun alone.

I'm happy that I've been successful on my diet for three days and also exercise at the health spa.

# Food fix

In the next journal entries I have hinted that I believe my problem is an addiction, akin to a smoking addiction, and I seek through prayer and meditation to understand it. This insight came with no knowledge of twelve-step programs and very little knowledge of addictions. I spent time each day seeking spiritual help in overcoming what I finally perceived to be a problem much bigger than myself.

<u>July 13, 1978</u>

Lately I've been having trouble staying on my diet. I've often had the whispering to pray for control as those trying to overcome other bad habits i.e. smoking etc. Today my mind was directed to the scripture in *Doctrine & Covenants* section 88 verse 119, which says, "Organize (yourself Ruth), prepare every needful thing."

I must organize my time so that I am not left with empty hours, which are the hours I fill with eating. That is the key to my success: organizing my time to know what I will be doing with it each minute.

Despite the spiritual insights into my food problem, I continued to be tormented with the compulsion to eat. With this compulsion came a spiral down into self-loathing and loss of self-esteem. This is succinctly described in a number of journal entries. I attempted in great detail to identify my problem times and then set out extensive and detailed plans to help me during such times. I must also note the context of this year: I was working full-time night shifts and suffering the effects associated with chronic sleep deprivation. This may also have contributed to the gloom and chaos in my food life.

July 24, 1978

Again I find myself having great difficulty in controlling my appetite and this is very grievous to me. When I lose control eating, I lose all self-respect. In fact, I turn into a first-rate slothful, dirty pig. I lose interest in my appearance, my character, and my work. I just get into an "I don't care about anything" mood. This is very depressing to me for I lose my sense of worth and value and it's all set off with overeating. I've been trying to identify what brings on my periods of compulsive eating.

As earlier mentioned, I felt that key to my eating problem was the scripture in *Doctrine and Covenants* 88: 119 where I am admonished to organize myself. I know I must plan every minute of my time in order to avoid compulsive eating.

Having identified some major problems, I now write new goals and guidelines for the next two months. These rules apply until October 9th.

1. no bread, cheddar cheese, graham or soda crackers—and no sugar in any form
2. plan on writing how to spend each day
3. fast for 24 hours each week

4. daily fifteen minute scripture ponder and prayer for strength to control appetite
5. never eat within four hours of sleeping
6. never eat alone
7. never eat when upset

All right, I feel prepared—I'm ready to start new with my goals and plans. Now it is Monday evening and I plan to fast until Thursday July 26th at noon, at which time I will drink one 8-oz glass of 2% skim milk. Then I will not eat again until 6:00 p.m., at which time I will have a fruit and boiled egg. Now, let me remember this always and every day. I will write you to tell you how I've done and feel about dieting.

# Goal writing disorder

In retrospect, I can see that many of my goals and plans for achievement of those goals were rather extreme routines and regimes that seemed doomed to failure. I was trying desperately to be perfect. Just looking at that plan makes me want to eat, even thirty years later! Despite such a lofty impossible regime, my moods temporarily soared on wings of hope for a miraculous transformation.

July 25, 1978

Today I feel great.

This evening I have been reading from Sterling Sill's book *Making the Most of Yourself*. I have been thrilled to learn of Ben Franklin's *Book of Virtues,* especially his statement re: temperance: "Eat not to dullness; drink not to elevation". Surely I have been guilty of the former—I also like his second virtue, silence. "Speak not but what may benefit others or yourself; avoid trifling conversation".

At present I feel great, having fasted well these past 24 hours, taking water only. I am confident that I can continue this until the set time.

It shouldn't come as a surprise that the confidence to maintain that lofty regime did not last. Four days later my journal records relapse again.

<u>July 29, 1978</u>

Yes, I have made mistakes in my eating.

I can clearly see now that I was very harsh with myself and held such stringent high expectations that I could only have maintained in a monastery on top a mountain in Tibet, praying without ceasing and having no access to food other than a crust of bread once a day. And yet, ever the optimist, I continued to pray and hope and diet and fast and look for the elusive miracle: that day when I would be happily thin and happily married.

<u>August 15, 1978</u>

Today in my prayers I have had a new thought. It makes me so happy when a new idea impresses on my mind. It is more important to be the right person than to find the right person. I know that I am not ready for I have not proven my ability in self-control. I know I must control my appetite before I am ready to marry.

Despite writing pages and pages of spiritual insights, strong desires, and lofty goals, food and weight continued to plague me for the remainder of that year I lived in Utah. It was time for a change in venue and menu. Certainly that would be the solution. So off I went back home again to Creston—always my secure spot safely nestled in the mountains of British Columbia.

# My big fat Canadian appetite

Be it ever so fattening, there's no place like home. That's where I always seemed to bungee back to for the security I sought in Creston. Back working in the Creston hospital, a number of colleagues commented on my increased size since leaving the previous year. "Where did that slim fit girl go that left here a year ago?" they asked. (Damn nurses—they notice everything!). Humiliated and ashamed, I boasted that I would soon be thin again, having just discovered another great diet to follow.

As the daily drudge of work routine set in, and I found myself still me, I started pining for a guy I met in Utah, wondering if I had left the one that might have been my rescuer from old-maid-hood and fat-hood. I had had only a few dates with him, but that was a few more dates than I had ever had in my entire 23 years. He had been a blind date set up by a woman I cared for on the maternity ward: her brother in law. Again, my insecurities with my body seemed to punctuate the journal entries covering my brief encounter with him. Though my weight is not recorded, I remember weighing in the range of 145 pounds – not exactly obese, but still feeling fat and awkward as recorded then.

<u>March 24, 1979</u>

I'll never forget that first glance of my blind date as he came through the door—blonde wavy hair and the most beautiful blue eyes I've ever seen. My mouth dropped open and I immediately became aware of my fat, my freckles, and my awkwardness. In short I felt like a toad and wished I could hide under the nearest bathtub.

Surprisingly, I survived that evening with relative ease—he showed slides of his mission. I smiled and nodded my head a lot. When I departed it was with the feeling that I would never see him again. I was totally deflated—felt horribly unattractive.

I did see him again. We had a bowling date. As above, all I recall is feeling fat and unattractive, awkward and inept at interacting with any semblance of normalcy. Alas it was the end of what never really started. I couldn't wait to leave the date and get home to eat my anxieties away. I guess I'd rather be eating.

And that's exactly what I did most of that winter living alone in an apartment in Creston.

As spring gave way to the summer of 1979, my angst over weight intensified and I set out another plan to beat it once and for all—another diet to end all diets. AGAIN! It seems that I felt that self-control was my problem and that life would be magically perfect if I could just get to the right weight. I did not seem to lack dreams or goal setting; they are both plentiful and recorded over and over again.

June 24, 1979

This gobb of girl called Ruth shall fast, except tomato juice, for the next three weeks. I am sick of having no control in my life—so much do I lack self-discipline. My number one problem is physical fat! I've got to get rid of it.

Only a day after this lofty recorded goal, I have recorded another mega food binge, yet I was still optimistic to overcome and still able to laugh at my endless, though poorly adhered to, plans.

June 25, 1979

Last night I ate everything that didn't run away from me (except the television set). Defeat? For one day, yes.

This morning I have not yet eaten, and am re-evaluating my hopes and dreams.

[10:00 PM] What hopes and dreams? DO NOT GIVE UP ON ME! I shall overcome—I shall become a model figure—a perfection body.

# I need a shrink!

Here in this next entry it seems that I am trying to psychoanalyze myself. Where's Freud when you need him? I really was trying hard to follow a plan, stars and all, and yet the harder I tried, the worse things became. The more I analyzed myself, using emotional, physical, and spiritual theories, the more confused and chaotic my food life and weight became.

June 26, 1979

Ruth has failed another day.

I bought a box of little sticky stars to mark the calendar for each successful day of dieting.

Sometimes I wonder just who I really am. It seems at times that some other person dwells within me – a conflicting person who doesn't want me to be the best that I can be. I sometimes don't know just what I want to be.

Perhaps I shall dwell for a moment on that—JUST WHO AM I? Number one, I am a human body with an immortal spirit. My spirit wants to be a super athletic, religious, beautiful, kind, lovable, charitable, patient perfect person. My body sometimes objects and perhaps forgets or does not know what it wants.

What I must learn is that in the eternities these two must function harmoniously. Therefore I must get them trained for this. Did you get that, body? Spirit is now in command. You must do as I say—hurt if you must, but don't quit.

June 27, 1979

Today I ate three eggs, a lot of cheese, bologna, bread, applesauce, milk, cream, peanut butter, and several servings of cake. Yuck! What a pig! This all happened before 3 p.m.

Then I went to work and ate nothing for the rest of the evening.

July 4, 1979

Would you believe that I have actually stuck to a sensible diet for three days now? I kid you not and I feel great!

July 8, 1979

Would you believe that I am on my eighth day of sticking strictly to a diet? Isn't it unbelievable? I've got seven stars on my calendar and will have my eighth when retiring tonight.

July 27, 1979

Today I managed to jog a mile and it felt great.

And off I jogged to try a new location to diet in.

## Girls just wanna be thin

After only a few months in Creston, again I had an urge to move on to somewhere else, to do something different than nursing, and to find a new location to find me.

In between the last entry and the next I impulsively decided to go to university in Lethbridge, Alberta, and get more education. I spent the summer making dresses to wear (making myself look slimmer was the plan). There was something about wearing dresses that gave me some confidence that people couldn't quite see my size. I can't quite explain such a phenomenon; it was just that way somewhere in my cerebral matter (probably a throwback to my childhood where dresses were the expectation).

Oddly, after only one day at university, I decided not to go. I was staying with my aunt in Cardston (about a 45 minute drive from Lethbridge) and stayed on to visit for a few weeks. While there, I developed a friendship with a guy, someone I had known for many years, but had not been romantically involved with before. I became totally enchanted with him and for a while it seemed to be a mutual attraction. In my journal I have recorded that he told me I was his idea of the ideal, the ultimate prize. It doesn't get much better than that! However, I also recall that he told me that he wanted me to lose a few pounds—the only change he would make to me. Immediately I launched on another diet to lose weight. I wasn't about to lose this opportunity for that eternal mate. Diet or die, I was prepared to be everything and anything he wanted me to be.

After a few blissful weeks with my presumed one and only, I returned to Creston to work while waiting to get a job in Alberta to be close to him. My exercise efforts stepped up as I was running on the high of love, certain that I would do anything to please the "one", even jog! It's an exercise I have never liked, but rather find revolting on so many levels, from the top of my scalp to the bottom of my soles.

The next journal entries are filled with the energetic high of presumed love. I could like myself now because a guy liked me. Pathetic as that seems it was the reality of my life then.

> October 13, 1979
>
> This past week I've been jogging every weekday morning.
>
> October 18, 1979
>
> It's great to be alive. This morning I was up at 6 a.m. and off jogging in my pale blue jogging suit.

The love affair with my self and with jogging came to a screeching and binging halt after a telephone conversation which turned out to be a formal rejection from my presumed one and only one. Food was there once again when rejection hit and I plunged myself into a litany of rejection lethargy and food vats, only to surface long enough to function in my job responsibilities.

Thankfully somewhere in my pity binge my bishop intervened and asked me to consider going on a full-time mission for the church. I heartily accepted his suggestion and it became the focus of my energies for the next few months, taking me through to the end of the year.

Early in 1980 I received an invitation to my presumed one and only's wedding, another terrible blow to my cellulite and sense of self. As recorded in this entry, I have vented a number of these feelings as well as reaffirming my craving to be beautiful.

<u>January 21, 1980</u>

Right now I feel bitter, used, discouraged—like I was just a fill-in for a bad month in his life.

I'd like to be one of the ten most beautiful women in the world. I'd like to go to a foreign country. This is probably what I'll do, for at present I am waiting for a mission call and hopefully I'll go to Hong Kong or Cambodia. Maybe I'll get run over by a tank (at least I'll be skinny).

I did go to Hong Kong and later to Thailand, where I worked with Cambodian refugees, and a new era of my life began. A couple months passed by before I record another litany of diet hopes. In the meantime I launched myself into another new world: the life of an LDS missionary.

# Mission impossible—converting fat to lean

On March 6, 1980 I entered the missionary training center in Provo, Utah for two months of Cantonese language training in preparation for a full time mission to Hong Kong. I was pumped and ready to be the ultimate disciplined missionary, complete with excellence in self-denial and sacrifice. Certainly my food-craving flesh would finally submit to the strength of my spirit.

Taken from a letter to my sister, I share my hopes for beating my weight problem while away from home for the next eighteen months.

March 29, 1980

One of my roommates is always receiving boxes of doughnuts, cookies, and cakes. She's skinny as a stick, eats sweets all the time, and has lost five pounds since she got here. There's no justice in this world. I live on lettuce, carrots, apples and such, blow myself into oblivion, and go down very slowly, but I'm not doing any crash dieting. I'm really eating quite well. I'm eating about eleven hundred calories daily and I think that if I lose only two pounds per month I'll still be really skinny when I return.

It wasn't long before I realized that I was still me, whether on a mission or not. I was still me with my food fears and issues. The next entry makes this clear and sets me on another goal-writing rampage. It's quite pathetic that as I entered the wonderful world of missionary service all I could think of is being thin when I returned home. Pathetic as it is, there it is recorded in my missionary journal. Even though I had other lofty and worthwhile goals, the weight thing superseded them all as number one.

April 5, 1980

I've just had one of my crave junk food attacks, so I am now gobbling fruit candy. I've come to the conclusion that I must write a few goals to accomplish by the end of my mission.

First, I want my mother to say, "You're too thin", and that is my first goal for my return home. To accomplish this goal I will hold to the following guidelines: I need to lose only two pounds per month, so here goes eleven hundred calories daily, excepting Sunday when I shall allow myself an extra three hundred. Of course this may need to be altered in Hong Kong. I hope to fit into size seven jeans when I return home.

The social culture of the missionary training center was such that new groups of missionaries arrived monthly while seasoned missionaries departed. Spiritual, emotional, and physical feasts typically accompanied these transitions. One such transition and accompanying feast is recorded in my journal.

April 6, 1980.

A fellow missionary and her companion had a party tonight. How ironic that I had just finished praying and asking God to help me control my appetite and not eat, then immediately following I went to a party and ate cake, pie, cookies and such, but I really enjoyed being with the departing group.

The spiritually focused environment of the missionary training center included daily speakers giving spiritual challenges. As recorded in the next entry, I took advantage of this spiritually saturated environment to once again seek divine assistance with my food problem. The next entry records details of a personalized prayer and plea to God.

April 13, 1980

Well tonight I accepted my mission leader's challenge to pray to God and say what I really feel and not use usual mechanical clichés. I prayed for about ten minutes and really let it all out, like I was talking to a good friend. It kind of felt good. I told Him my concern over my weakness of gobbling unnutritious foods. Well, He said that He can turn weaknesses into strengths if I try sincerely to do so. I'm really going to try. I want the healthiest body possible, and then my spirit will be happier too. This is exciting. He promised me that I really can have great strength in resisting junky food, the gooey's, chocolate etc., but I must give it all my effort as well.

Perhaps I never did figure out what really was all my effort and as such never fully engaged myself to conquer with the help of God. Perhaps I lacked faith and what I lacked in faith I made up for in writing and ruminating on weight woes. The very thin missionary I mentioned in the letter to my sister continued to be an anomaly to me. I envied her thin lithe body and her approach to food. She never gave a thought to what she ate.

I wanted to be her. I wanted to be free from the obsession as much as I wanted to be free from the fat. I mention this skinny missionary in the next couple journal entries

<u>May 2, 1980</u>

This evening a fellow missionary and I went out running around the missionary training center and had a great heart to heart talk. She's a super person and I can't admire her enough. She's kind to everyone. I think she's near to being what I imagine an angel is like in character. Besides that, she's got a gorgeous slender body that I covet daily. Ha! And she covets my brain. I want my body to be as slim as hers when I return home from my mission.

<u>May 5, 1980 [In flight to Hong Kong]</u>

My favourite skinny missionary is sitting beside me and just said, "If we ate as much spiritually as we do physically, we would be spiritual giants."

That's easy for her to say. She's not fat!

# Whither thou goest I will go, whatever thou eatest, I will eat

In early May I landed in Hong Kong filled with hope and fear and food and anticipation for what the next sixteen months would bring. Most of all, I hoped that being in a foreign country would change me and I would no longer eat to excess. I hoped that those skinny little Chinese women would rub off on me and that I would become them, at least in body.

It didn't take long to realize that I was me, even in Hong Kong. Damn it! I went half way around the world and there I was. It was still me with my food orgies front and center. Soon after landing I was, you guessed it, planning my next diet, albeit, my **first** one in Hong Kong.

Fortunately, or unfortunately, I shared an apartment with other food confused missionaries and we bonded over food. We commiserated with each other, the fat white women who couldn't possibly understand the thin Chinese women. My thin buddy from the missionary training center was sent to the island of Macau far from me and I did not see her for many months. I missed her. I wanted to be her. Instead I was me and I was companioned with a portly American woman who loved to eat. She ate more than I did and she shared her ubiquitous treats generously. I loved her but I hated her more.

### May 17, 1980 Hong Kong

My missionary companion and I bought digestive cookies and ginger snaps for lunch today and made ourselves sick. We've decided to eat everything we want until June 1st then go on a diet and get thin for area conference in October.

### May 27, 1980

Yesterday we, meaning me and my fellow missionaries, ate everything in our paths: cheerios, corn flakes, peanut butter, bread, sugar, worms, cheese etc. Finally, we were utterly disgusted with ourselves and decided to all go on a diet to get these gross bodies in shape. Today we drank water all day – no food. I have a slight headache but last night I had a headache from eating too much.

This sounds like a broken record already and I am really only getting started. The cycle of dieting and binging continues as well as the highs and lows of moods, still correlating inversely with the numbers on the scale. The next few journal entries focus again on my quest for thinness and for the ultimate solution to my problem

### June 19, 1980

I feel good about myself in the area of appetite. I've had great control these past few days and feel it's very important for my spiritual as well as physical well-being.

### June 20, 1980

I really want to excel. I want an excellent healthy slim body.

From a missionary notebook recording thoughts and quotes from numerous conferences, I have recorded the following quote attributed to the wife of a visiting church authority.

June, 1980

It's not what you eat but what is eating you that causes the problem.

This quotation has so much more meaning to me now than it did over thirty years ago as a young adult in a foreign mission. I agree that what is eating me is the problem because whatever it is that is eating me is causing me to eat and eat and eat and eat and this just eats me up more and more and the problem goes round and round and round again. It's a perplexing philosophical question that has no answer. Which came first, the eating or being eaten?

June 23, 1980

I wondered why the Chinese women are so thin if they eat so much greasy food. I asked an elderly Chinese woman who said that it's because after each meal the Chinese people drink some kind of hot vegetable soup which chases the food thru the body and prevents fat. Great Honk! If it's true, I must get the magic recipe.

July 4, 1980

A fellow missionary is halfway thru her mission today so she made chocolate cake to celebrate. I ate some and felt rather sick because of its sweetness. More and more I realize the importance of physical health and how closely it is related to spiritual and emotional health. I have felt great these past couple weeks that

I've really been controlling my physical appetite and when we walk a lot, I even feel better.

# Life's a binge then you diet

As before mission life, I continued to set near impossible goals for myself and continued to bounce between the agony of binging and the ecstasy of control.

> July 23, 1980
>
> I fasted today, being that I've really been in a slump this past week. That loss of control I so hate has been the pits lately. I am now back in control, praise the beasts and cockroaches. I'm hungry but it's a better feeling than sour stomach due to over gorging on everything that doesn't run. As before mentioned, my number one goal for this mission is to get control over my flesh and get rid of all excess fat. I'm going to weigh less than 110 pounds when I return home in September 1981.

Less than 110 pounds!? It seems that, while I was losing no weight, I was definitely losing my mind. Being around all those perennially petite Chinese women was skewing my image of what should be normal. I now wanted to be as tiny as they were. Extreme starving accompanied my extreme desire as recorded in this next journal entry.

### July 25, 1980

As written on our thought board in the apartment I have copied: "Your life is influenced more by your own thoughts and desires than anything else." Well I'm going to dwell on this desire to be slim and fit. I continue to fast to show God really how much I really want what I am at present praying for. I'm exercising faith thru fasting for four days – water only. I know God grants according to faith. Well, there's not a whole lot of things I want so much as to fast four days and it is a rather difficult thing when all around are eating snacks. My fellow missionary is forever buying snacks, giving me little gobby gooey stuff to eat, but I've just tucked it away out of sight for I have a desire that means far more to me than four days of food.

### July 27, 1980

Being that our missionary apartment was in charge of lunch last night we hustled around making cookies but you know I never took one bite. They smelled great, but I remembered my commitment to God and controlled myself. A former church president has said something like, the greatest strength comes when we conquer the flesh, and today again I have successfully gone without food even though I have been surrounded by all kinds of goodies. The joy of self-discipline far surpasses the bit of pleasure from overeating—especially gobby sweets.

Somewhere in my nutrient-starved brain I grossly misinterpreted sensible counsel from wise men. I'm sure that conquering the flesh did not mean to starve it to death! More evidence of my all-or-nothing approach to life. Predictably no one (except maybe a wacko on a hunger strike) can keep up that regime for long and the next entry records the fall as well as more extreme goals.

<u>July 31, 1980</u>

After teaching a lesson, my fellow missionary and I escaped for a few minutes to the Victoria Park and ate ice-cream together. I felt rather like a criminal but at the same time it was a much needed fifteen minute TIME-OUT break. Last night my fellow missionary and I decided that when we return home she will weigh 118 pounds and I will weigh 108 pounds. These are our passwords from now on.

It looks like I had a few months reprieve from writing about my food obsession as I struggled with the challenges of being a missionary in a foreign land. It was hot. It was humid. I was homesick. I ate my way through the summer. It seemed a better option than giving up and going home. Late summer finds me returning once again to the obsession of food and weight.

<u>Sept. 2, 1980</u>

When this mission is over I'm going to fall into my mother's arms and cry incessantly and unceasingly for several hours. Hopefully by then my weight will be such that I won't break her arms. This really is national self-pity week.

<u>Sept. 16, 1980</u>

I am frustrated, depressed, lonely, and eating myself into oblivion. I just don't know what's wrong with me. It's like I've lost all control of my own life and I feel rather desperate.

<u>Sept. 19, 1980</u>

Maybe I'll starve myself to death or at least to illness. Ha! But you know this motor mouth. There's no danger of me starving myself. I'll probably eat myself to death instead.

I was rather melodramatic with my food fantasies and failures. O diet, where is thy sting!

# Moon cake, moon face

Hong Kong introduced me to the delectably delicious moon cake. I couldn't get enough of them and ate them with the gusto of someone who knew she would never see them again. It is no surprise then that these amazing seasonal treats are mentioned in my journal.

<u>Sept. 20, 1980</u>

Tonight I am eating another deliciously fattening moon cake. They are truly delightful and I have to get my fill before the holiday season ends, for I will not be in Hong Kong this time next year to eat them again.

With the continuation of compulsive eating, I again try to diagnose and understand this perplexing and complex problem as recorded in numerous journal entries.

<u>Sept. 23, 1980</u>

I feel so fortunate so there's no reason for me to be depressed and eat myself into oblivion. So why am I? Perhaps it's the fault of my hormones.

In my desperation seeing the months fly by and the pounds pack on, I drafted an affidavit and swore with an oath that I would eat only a thousand calories per day for the remainder of my mission (still twelve months to go). I had my companion sign it with me and another missionary witness it. I was sure this would seal my fate and be the clincher for success. Alas, it just perpetuated more guilt and eating.

<u>Sept. 26, 1980</u>

I really don't know what's wrong with me. I feel like I've degenerated rapidly these past few weeks. Every day I've eaten myself into oblivion, awakened feeling ill from food overdose, and the first thing I do is start stuffing food in my mouth. I feel that I've got to hit a turning point somewhere or hit rock bottom so I can start back up again.

What a pain! I feel like I've gained twenty pounds in the last two weeks. At this rate I'll weigh a ton when I get home next year and that's the last thing I want. When I get off the plane in Cranbrook I want to be less than 110 pounds, super skinny with shoulder length hair and a big confident smile on my face. I'll just be a gorgeous bone structure.

I think I better use this time to reassess and recommit my hopes for the end of my mission. It's a third over and I'm no nearer my weight goal than I was when I started. I've had great success for a month then went on a binge and gained it all back.

I will start again on Monday, September 29th – and I really mean it. I'm going to eat no more than a thousand calories daily and fast every P-day [missionary day off] and I'm going to stick with it until I've lost all my excess weight. This is getting ridiculous. I'm sick of being this fat slothful ugly person and I'm going to change before I return home eleven months from now. I know there will be terribly rough times when I'm frustrated, unhappy, and hungry, but I'm not going to turn to food anymore. I'll cry in the bathroom or I'll write in here or lose myself in a good daydream. I can't go on being this fat, lazy, undesirable creep.

I know that if I'm fat when I go home, it will just destroy the excitement of it all and I'll not want anyone to see me. I've got to prepare now to make that day great. My life is such a series of up and down cycles. Sometimes I've got such great control, nothing could make me overeat. Then other times nothing can stop me from eating. There are times that I am so disciplined in study, exercise, prayer, work, and appetite. All aspects seem to really affect each other. It seems that if I fail in one, the others soon follow the failure pattern.

Goodnight from FAT, FAT, the water Rat.

Nov. 10, 1980

I can't wait to be slim but that too takes time and teaches me patience.

Nov. 17, 1980

I celebrated my certification in Cantonese language so I am afraid to say that I broke my written commitment of November 6th but hope to get back with it from now and hereafter to skinniness.

Nov. 18, 1980

I sometimes feel like a stranger to myself, like I'm standing off in the distance watching myself functioning and in many ways myself destroying me while I stand by and watch with terror.

Nov. 20, 1980

I feel so self-defeated from so many commitments broken, so many goals un-reached.

What has become of me? What have I done with those goals of so long ago? The time has come and gone. So many months have gone by and I have not accomplished a thing and have not become the slightest bit closer to my mission goals.

It's time to shake off the sloth within me, get the fat out, and fly.

Nov. 24, 1980

A fellow missionary and I went jogging tonight. It just about killed me. I am so out of shape. I coughed, choked, and vomited. My lungs are just burning. There are so many muscles I've not used for so long and they're probably full of car exhaust, smog, etc. and TB.

December 1st, 1980

Wt. 152 pounds. Gross.

I look at that last entry and think, it's all relative really. At this point in my life I would be quite happy to weigh 152 pounds. Back then at age 25 it seemed like the ultimate shame and torture.

The weight saga continued as I made more attempts to console my tormented soul.

Dec. 2, 1980

I am a real yoyo—and I wonder why this is the case. Why do I go from such exceeding highs to such lows and self-degradation in only a matter of hours? In some ways I feel I have lost my self-respect because of my extreme lack of control and willpower to stick to my commitments.

<u>December 8, 1980</u>

Wt. 155 pounds. Gross.

I can only guess that the end-of-year attitude prevailed and I caved totally to the food demons. But once again a new year dawns with high hopes for achieving the ultimate dream, being thin.

<u>Jan. 1, 1981</u>

Well, I guess being New Year's Day we're expected to set resolutions, goals, or whatever for the New Year. It's strange to think that I will be home this year and I definitely want to make 1981 my year for shaping up physically. I suppose every overweight female in the universe makes this same New Year's resolution.

The anxiety over weight increases as my mission months steadily wind down and I see other missionaries heading home. Three weeks into the New Year and I am still me, only a fatter more anxious me.

<u>Jan. 25, 1981</u>

I've just got over seven months to go and I'm no closer to reaching my goal of April 3rd than I was when I wrote it. It makes me think of a fellow missionary. About four months ago she said that she was going to be a skinny fox when she goes home. Well, she goes home next week and she's not quite that skinny fox. She looks rather like she did four months ago. So I think, "The harvest is over, my mission ended, and I am still fat". But I've got time to change all that.

Jan. 26, 1981

This afternoon we had to go out for some errands and go to the bank and inevitably ended up at the Dairy Creamery for ice-cream. This is a disgrace to the glutton race.

The dreaded camera catches me fat and center. I can't believe what I see and now turn to a thin missionary for help. Still, as further entries evidence, I continued to self-destruct with food.

Feb. 5, 1981

I had my picture taken wearing the traditional Sung Dynasty costume. Here it is and I'm grossly obese. I had a good talk with a fellow missionary about my obesity and she's going to behavior modify me. I need it. I sure need something. I'm just getting fatter and fatter and more miserable. Look at that gross face. It must weigh a ton itself.

Feb. 6, 1981

My stomach has been terribly upset today from the candy I overdosed on yesterday.

Feb. 7, 1981

I am so fat, it's just gross. If I had thought a year ago that I would be this fat this year, I would likely have jumped in the pond with a lead weight around my neck.

Again, I was rather melodramatic about my seemingly astronomical problem!

# A time to lose

Between the last entry and the next, I was transferred in March to the Thailand mission to work in refugee camps near Phanat Nikom. I was very excited to get out of the crowded noisy busyness of Hong Kong. As soon as I arrived in Thailand I felt a tremendous relief and immediately started losing weight. It was like a huge emotional and physical weight was lifted from me. I was certain to be thin in time for my return to Canada in the fall. This next entry was about six weeks after arriving in Thailand.

<u>April 27, 1981</u>

Today I was humored by a remark of one of our refugee translators. First thing this morning he said, "Ruth, have you adjusted to the weather here and Thai food?" I laughed and said, "Why do you ask?" He said, "You are not getting weight. Getting skinny." I laughed more—what a delight! That's just the remark a hungry dieter longs to hear.

It also helped in Thailand that I lived with several missionaries who wanted to jog and take care of themselves. They were a great motivation and for a few months I rode the wave of weight loss, happily soaking up all the compliments about my diminishing girth.

May 13, 1981

About myself, I feel good. I feel like I do have control of myself and am learning a lot of self-discipline through jogging.

May 18, 1981

I really have to chuckle because my mission leaders are so worried that I'm too thin and must be sick. They think they need to make me eat more. It's kind of nice to be greeted with, "You're too thin". I like it and I'm not going to eat excessively to please anyone. My mission president's wife prepared a beautiful dinner of ham, scalloped potatoes, and candy pineapple for us. Now that I've become known as being a super willpower person, it really helps to have all eyes on me to see what I will do in the situation of being faced with a gorgeous big meal. Well, I stood the test and ate a tiny portion of potato and a large serving of string beans with some plain fresh pineapple, which was served beside the candy pineapple. I love the feeling of self-control. With each success at self-control my willpower doubles. It feels great.

May 19, 1981

I know that I have gone through times when I've really disliked myself because of lack of self-discipline and then I became sloppy with no care about appearance, lazy, and really ugly. But those times are in the past. At present I feel so good about myself and I feel my appearance and countenance and actions towards others are much more attractive.

The reality of day to day life and eating still presented itself, even in Thailand where I had had such success with food control. The house I lived in with other missionaries was looked after by a Thai woman who, despite language difficulties, became my coach, conscience, and confidante. Her attempts to help me and keep me honest are recorded in this next entry.

<u>June 21, 1981</u>

Lately, our Thai maid has been coaching me on being slim. Her advice is to eat "rice, no fat", she says, but "potato fat, butter, fat". One night last week my fellow missionaries and I had an ice-cream and cookie party. The next morning our maid said, "If you keep eating ice-cream you get fat."

Somehow the maid's advice sunk in and got me quickly back on track so as to avoid a complete derailment into the abyss of food hell. Now into July, I was still on a slim high. I have not recorded my weight during this wonderful euphoric state, but I do recall a day when I stepped on the scale and it registered 129 pounds. For me it was a virtual step into the Promised Land.

<u>July 3, 1981</u>

Life is really a lot more enjoyable when you're slim. I think it is. I like myself a lot more when I'm slim.

Even all these years later, I still like myself better when I'm slim--mer!

# A time to gain

The wonderful weight euphoria of Thailand ended abruptly with my transfer, in late July, to the Philippine Island of Palawan where, with one other missionary, we initiated a teaching program in the refugee camps there. Unlike the transition from Hong Kong to Thailand, which was a huge relief, this transition proved to be more stressful and challenging. I felt overwhelmed with the responsibilities now placed on me. Food once again became my drug of choice for assuaging the anxiety I felt.

July 25, 1981

For the past few days I have eaten myself sick every blasted day. There is a terrible wave of gorging and depression settling in as I quickly pile on the fat I have worked so hard to lose these past few months.

I know I feel rather at a loss of identity here. It's like I've been untimely ripped from my security in Panat Nikom and I must face a drastic change all alone.
I certainly cannot understand why this throws my eating pattern off so drastically. I guess food is the one thing I feel secure with.

Somewhere in Palawan I found a book on sugar, which I have no recall of except that it is mentioned in this next journal entry. Along with it I once again commit to swear off sugar.

Now nearing the end of my mission, my goals have modified somewhat to a more reachable scope.

<u>July 26, 1981</u>

I've just been reading a rather frightening book on the effects of sugar in our bodies. Yikes! I know that I feel terrible, sluggish, depressed, and irritable when I eat too much sugar. I would like to go completely off sugar. Perhaps I will try this as a trial for the remainder of my mission. I have about ten weeks left to go before I go home.

Sometimes I am frightened that my mission time is almost over and I am not quite molded into that person I want to be when I return home. Perhaps my greatest desire is to have a healthy, physically fit slim body because with this control and slimness comes a great sense of self-respect, self-confidence, big smiles, and just well-rounded friendliness.

So then this is a time to reflect and re-evaluate, to recommit and rejuvenate my desires to be of optimum health. I no longer want to be an absolute underweight stick. All I want is to be the normal weight for my height and to have good muscle tone and be in good physical condition.

First, I simply must STOP eating garbage, especially sugar to start with.

As recorded in this next entry, I had discovered the wonderful mood elevating properties of exercise and quickly descended into a low mood without it. The wonderful routine of jogging with other missionaries in Thailand now became a thing of the past. As an LDS missionary being alone is not allowed, so a missionary is dependent on what her companion is willing to do, sort of like having a spouse that you can't get away from.

July 31, 1981

Jogging gave me such an emotional strength and self-mastery as I have not experienced previously. This past month I have degenerated rapidly—no jogging, no self-control in eating, just gorge and sleep. I am ashamed and far from happy like the happiness I experienced through jogging and sensible eating.

August 1, 1981

My companion couldn't jog this morning, so I did some skipping alone. Not a whole lot but just enough to realize how degenerate my state of fitness is. There has to be a beginning again somewhere so it might as well be here with a few skips. I've got only nine weeks here. I've got to get the most out of this place with each passing day.

Nine weeks is still nine weeks and I've got some pounds to re-lose before I am seen by everyone. I wonder why I even bother to lose weight, I just gain it back. What a depressing cycle it is.

In the next entry, I once again compare myself to an alcoholic with my self-defeating behavior. The self-hatred is palpable as well as the frustration with self. Finding a routine in Palawan proved to be a bigger challenge than anticipated.

August 3, 1981

This morning my fellow missionary and I made a feeble attempt at jogging. Do you want to know how far I made it? About one minute. My pants are tight, my abdomen protruding, and my breasts pendulous. This decay of fitness has all happened in just one month. When July opened, I was fifteen pounds lighter than now. I was jogging four miles and I felt superb except for a sore throat. I'm ashamed of myself. Why did I work so hard for months to lose weight and then in such a short time I've put it all back on? It's despicable! And I feel particularly rotten because I ate a bunch of ice-cream and crud yesterday. I feel like alcoholics must feel with their self-defeating behavior.

August 13, 1981

I am not slim like I wanted to be. I have gained back several pounds and am now not slim, but I would like to be on my return.

More than a month passed in Palawan and I had still not managed to capture self-control again. I loved the refugees and spent long hours with them. I wanted to rescue all of them and felt a deep sadness that they should suffer so much and continue to suffer when I could go home to the peace, freedom, and security of Canada. I gave them all I could both emotionally and financially yet continued to struggle within myself, focusing on me and my weight problem.

September 5, 1981

I really don't know why I've become such a degenerate here. I am on a beautiful tropical island teaching refugees and really loving it, and yet within myself I feel utter despair, loneliness, and a strange emptiness that I am trying to fill with food, but it's not working.

## September 6, 1981

My money is at an all-time low because of my generosity to the refugee cause, yet I continue to eat. Perhaps I will come to the point of no eating through necessity. I hope so. Then I'll lose some fat. This is an eternal pain for me—lose weight, gain it back, lose weight, gain it back, lose, gain, lose, gain, gain, gain. I'm sick of it. Whenever I'm in an emotional knot or any depression, my first instinct is eat, eat, and eat. Why do I turn to food every time anything goes wrong or goes right?

There is no mention of weight problems again in the last couple months of my mission. I arrived home in November, 1981. One of the first things I did was weigh myself and found that I was 138 pounds—slimmer than when I had left, but not the 110 pounds I had dreamed about and written about in numerous journal entries in four foreign countries, as well as flights over the ocean. My mother didn't tell me I was too thin, damn it!

It was now time for the next chapter in my life, post-mission.

# Feed me. Feed me not.

In the months following my return to Canada, I once again worked as a nurse in the Creston Hospital and began dating a man I had known prior to my overseas mission. Within a few months, I had once again focused on my weight and concerns over appearance. Even though I had attracted the attention of an eligible professional in my home town, I was despairing once again over my lack of control over food. Having a man in my life did not magically solve my self-loathing problems. In short, I was still me, still recording my attempts to be beautiful and slim, and still measuring myself against impossible standards.

March 21, 1982

Let me dwell on another depressing subject: my appearance. Again I am a shambles—gaining weight, pants too tight, belly rolling over waist, and the list goes on. There are times I'd give almost anything to be slim. Now I reflect back to June of last year when I was slender and so fit. I know I can do it again, but sometimes I feel like, why should I even go through all the hassle of losing weight when nine times out of ten I'll gain it right back on? Just the thought of it makes me want to eat.

I'm a pig, snort, but I know I can lose and keep slim if I'm always motivated to do it.

I lived out 1982, my usual neurotic food freak, still feeling fat as the New Year approached and recording fat highlights from the New Year's Eve party I attended.

January 3, 1983 Re: New Year's Eve party.

I felt ugly because I had a big pimple on my face and I felt fat.

January 14, 1983

My moods are up one day and down the next and sometimes I simply don't care about myself. Other times I'm ultra-disciplined. Today I'm a slob.

As life unfolded I realized the challenges of developing and maintaining a romantic relationship and interacting with the emotional ups and downs of others. From my journal recordings it seems that I had my own set of emotional ups and downs and felt overwhelmed with those of another person. So what did I do? You guessed it—eat!

February 19, 1983

I can't take his depression any longer. It drags me down too much. My sister made some cookies and we gorged on them.

As the next entry indicates, I managed to lose some weight during the winter. I don't recall exactly how that was done, except perhaps my usual semi-starvation dieting. With a wedding coming up, I was likely motivated to look good and slim for the big day.

March 5, 1983

I put on the burgundy cords I bought at Christmas. Much to my surprise they are quite a bit too big to wear now. It's nice to have lost that much weight, but not nice to be out an expensive pair of pants.

# 'Til diet do we part

I married on April 1, 1983. I know! I know! It was April fool's day, but it was also Good Friday so that should have helped right? Typically when the much anticipated weight loss event was over, the weight gain started again. Alas, I was still me, married or not. I carried me wherever I went.

Whatever happened to that fantasy I had that marriage would make me suddenly whole and free of excess weight and food obsession and lumps and bumps and thighs? What a shocker that was! Married or single, I was still me and that sucked as far as I was concerned. The attention of a man did not give me the completeness I fantasized about. Looking for myself in someone else did not give me the me I dreamed about.

Within months of marrying I was once again setting weight loss goals. The weight loss magic was gone, the fat was back, and my clothes no longer fit.

<u>July 24, 1983</u>

Weekly goals:

1. *follow yoga 28 day plan*
2. *eat only natural foods—no sugar*
3. *go for ½ hour brisk walk daily*

I'm not sure how those goals panned out, but I am guessing not well, certainly not lasting. During this time I continued to work full-time shift work as a nurse. My journal is void of weight and food issues for a few months, not even New Year's goals discuss them. The year ended and a new one began without me journaling about my size and food issues. The next entry indicates that I have still not solved my problem. It also records my indestructible and unstoppable optimism that I will overcome.

<u>February 23, 1984</u>

A new year is now well upon me and I've not rectified my slothfulness. Isn't it great to have a new day dawn every 24 hours to start again?

You gotta love optimism like that.

# Binging for two

In the summer of 1984 I became pregnant with my first child. What a relief it was to abandon dieting and eat. I was in girl heaven. No diets. No measuring food. No counting calories. Just big clothes and big appetite. The following entry makes reference to dieting before this time.

> October 7, 1984
>
> When I discovered I was pregnant I was a bit worried because I had been dieting and drinking a fair amount of diet Fresca and thought it may have done some harm.

I recall being extremely relieved that I was pregnant and had an excuse not to diet. The forks were out, the plates were filled, there was no calorie barred, and I was on an eating rampage of epic proportions. As the pounds packed on, I started again fantasizing about being slim. There is something exhilarating about knowing that the diet does not have to start for several months. Having the discipline tucked away in the future gives a false sense of security while eating and planning for the months ahead.

Books on visualization seemed to be everywhere during this time and I gulped them down with the same enthusiasm that I gulped my food. At last I would be slim by creating a picture in my mind of what I wanted to be. All I had to do to succeed was to see it. Life was getting better all the time with my new-found books on visualization.

December 8, 1984

I am creating a mental picture of something I have wanted for a long time and that is a slender fit lithe body. I'm going to reach this goal by my 30th birthday. This is the picture I will keep in mind daily.

I visualized and chanted myself into a frenzy of change. As I packed on the pounds I faithfully chanted my new found mantra, 'I am lean; I am light; I am long'. Certainly such mantras and mental exercises would counterbalance the calories I was stuffing into my face. Ah, the sweet joy of fantasy and denial!

After a weight gain of 53 pounds, my first child was born on February 26, 1985, a lovely little girl weighing only six pounds three ounces named Joan Nicole. I had reached an all-time high in my weight and simply accepted that it would not last. I would get it off and more, and become the slim person I wanted to be. As a breastfeeding mother I did not diet, but started walking regularly to get the excess weight off.

May 31, 1985

I've been walking 3½ miles daily for a while now, usually in the early morning after Joan's breakfast. She sleeps through the night until about 5 or 6 a.m. After she eats I put her in her snugly carrier on my chest and we go walking. I feel so good out walking in the fresh morning air. I think out a lot of frustration and anger. By the time I've finished my walk I always feel better about my life as it is.

Though not much is recorded during that year of caring for a baby, I recall feeling like breastfeeding was absolutely magic for weight loss. I seemed to eat what I wanted and counted on breastfeeding and walking to burn it off. I had a daily mantra: nine months to get up, nine months to get down. Overeating continued to be a challenge but I seemed to balance the calorie intake with walking and breastfeeding.

<u>January 12, 1986</u>

I am going to write down a few of my coming week goals. Walk 3½ miles daily Mon-Fri.

<u>January 22, 1986</u>

Sometimes I wonder why I ever bother to set a bunch of goals then never meet them. I guess it makes me feel like I'm doing something at least by writing them down.

<u>February 14, 1986</u>

I made some boiled chocolate cookies for a Valentine treat but ate too many as usual and now I feel like a blob.

<u>April 17, 1986</u>

I made my 4½ mile walk in sixty minutes today. I feel so good physically and I love my daily walk out in the fresh spring air.

I end this diet phase on a positive note, enjoying mothering my baby and living, for the most part, a food balanced life, happily breastfeeding my precious daughter until months into pregnancy number two in the fall of 1986.

# Too much on my plate

During my second pregnancy I once again started gaining rapidly, relieved to not have to diet. Pregnancy was a food free-for-all and I relished it with great excitement. As the weight piled on at record speed however, I became alarmed, knowing that the twenty pounds I had piled on already could not possibly be explained by a six inch fetus. As much as I fantasized that my little six inch super zygote could be floating around in ten gallons of amniotic fluid and nourished by a ten pound placenta, I could not deny that the weight was sitting smack dab on my expanding derriere and had nothing to do with fetal growth.

I was gaining so fast that my then husband (a veterinarian and farmer) pointed out to me that his steers in the feedlot couldn't gain that fast. Things were getting fatter than expected and I became alarmed. I would have to face the fat sooner or later, so why not take a proactive approach and get help? This was my first attempt to manage weight by seeking professional help.

> November 24, 1986
>
> I am now seeing the hospital dietician weekly on referral from my doctor. When I saw him last week I asked for a referral to her to prevent my gaining any more weight during the last four months of my pregnancy. I've already gained more than I should and I feel too

fat. I don't want to go through the gross fat I went through last time. I've had one visit with the dietician now and feel much better already. I'm optimistic and feel in control for the time being.

November 26, 1986

I went to the dietician. I enjoy going there. I lost 1 ½ pounds so I was doubly pleased. I guess all this raw cabbage eating is paying off.

As with all my dieting attempts, the success was short lived. CABBAGE?! Seriously, how long could that last? And with another infernal Christmas season coming on, what could I do but eat? Besides that, the dietician wasn't available through the holidays, so what was a pregnant dieter to do? Eat! The next entry records the food rut and fall out of Christmas binging. What the hell was I doing milking a cow by hand, or by any means for that matter?

January 6, 1987

It's so hard to get out of a slothful rut. I've been quite a slob over the holidays and am finding it difficult to get out and milk the cow in the morning. I'm packing more weight now and feeling quite clumsy. Tomorrow I go to see the dietician after not being for almost a month. I know I've packed on some excess weight in the past month.

January 7, 1987

I went to the dietician today. I gained seven pounds in the past month. I suppose it could have been worse.

January 21, 1987

I went to see the dietician this morning. I am gaining, but not at a horrific rate. I did the horrific gaining in the first five months. Ah well, I must fight that off after delivery.

In a journal written to my baby, I have recorded some references to my burgeoning weight and hopes that he is gaining it rather than me.

February 15, 1987

Dear Baby,

I saw the doctor last week. He says that you are not a big baby. Why not? Certainly I feed you plenty. At least I feed myself plenty. Isn't it getting through to you? I'd rather you gain than me.

My second child, Marshall Lee, was born on March 22, 1987. Despite my attempts to combat weight-gain during the pregnancy, I still managed to gain more than I had with my first child. One bonus was that my son weighed almost two pounds more than my daughter had weighed at birth. Woohoo! That meant two less pounds for me to lose. Even during the pain of labor, I commented on my size when the nurse asked if I wanted a mirror to see the delivery as it happened.

March 22, 1987

The nurse asked me if it would bother me to have the mirror set up so I could see the delivery. I said that the only thing that would bother me about it would be to see the size of my butt exposed in full.

Is it just me or is there something wrong with a woman who can fret about her butt size during the most intense pain and agony of labor? What about the neurotic state of a mother who can think of her newborn's weight in terms of her needs, then records that in a letter to her newborn? Was I sick or what?

In a journal written to my son, I have mentioned his weight and what it meant to me.

March 22, 1987

Dear Marshall,

Thank God you're here and a boy. You were born at 8:25 this morning and at this time are four hours old. I am very thrilled with you, that you are a boy and that you weigh eight pounds. That means I'll weigh less.

With my son barely two weeks old, I was feeling the angst of getting the weight off, planning again to breastfeed and walk it off as I had done two years earlier.

April 8, 1987

I haven't started an exercise routine yet but hope to get walking soon. I'm anxious to get losing fat.

April 13, 1987

Today I finally forced myself to get out and do my walk routine. I've got to get into walking or I'll not get rid of my excess weight.

May 22, 1987

I've been walking regularly for six weeks now, 4-5 days a week, first thing in the morning. I must be getting into shape. I feel good. I saw the dietician on Wednesday and weighed in. It was about what I expected, but I feel good.

June 7, 1987

My favorite hours of the day are between 5 and 8 a.m. I get up and feed Marshall, then we go out for an hour walk. I push him in the stroller. When we get back home I take him out with me and milk the cow. I feed the cattle and chickens and I always feel like I've accomplished so much before breakfast.

As I read these journal entries and reflect on the stress of my life during those years of trying to be super mom, super wife, super farmer, super everything, I marvel that I did not eat even more to cope with the overwhelming tasks I felt required to do. Just thinking about it now makes me want to dive into a vat of ice-cream! No wonder I had so many days of excess food to cope with the excess responsibilities in my life.

July 25, 1987

Friday evening we made raspberry ice-cream and chocolate chip cookies. I overate.

I continued to see the dietician for a few months and felt motivated by my weekly sessions with her.

September 2, 1987

I went into town to see the dietician. I lost 1½ pounds ☒.

September 9, 1987

I went to the dietician this afternoon and am down to 143 pounds.

September 15, 1987

I'm not looking forward to being weighed tomorrow after eating popcorn and peanuts and chocolate chip cookies tonight.

September 16, 1987

Teeheeheehee! My weight is down 1 ¼ pounds. I'm so pleased with myself.

I'm feeling good about my appearance lately. I can fit into most of my clothes comfortably.

September 22, 1987

I've had so much sugar these past few days. I've been a dreadful pig.

September 23, 1987

My overeating finally caught up with me: weight up by two pounds today—Eek! Can I hope that it is water retention?

Last night we had some of our fresh trout for supper then made strawberry ice-cream. I felt like a bloated heifer. I've really got to stop this overindulging soon before I balloon out and look like I'm gaining instead of losing. It must be PMS that's doing this to me.

September 29, 1987

I feel blue today, just blue. I want to eat sweets and generally do nothing, which is difficult to do with two small children. It must be PMS or something. I'm just blue.

Look at these measurements! They're pretty impressive for me, having a baby and breastfeeding and all. I wish I had those measurements now.

October 7, 1987

This morning I went to see the dietician. My weight is down 2½ pounds. Hurray!

Measurements: 36" bust

26½" waist

37¼" hip

23" thigh

October 8, 1987

I made a pan of midnight mints to give my husband's hairdresser for his birthday tomorrow. I'm so proud of myself because I did not take one bite of it—not even so much as a lick of the spoon!

For a brief period I seemed to have things all together within myself and my cellulite. I was flying high as summer turned to fall and another birthday rolled around.

October 9, 1987 32nd birthday

I feel, for the first time in my life, that I am in control of myself physically. I am eating, drinking, and exercising sensibly and in balance with my body's needs. I feel at peace with my body.

# Irritable binge syndrome

Just when I thought things were under control, something flipped me out of sugar sync again.

October 27, 1987

I'm not looking forward to my weigh in tomorrow because I've been eating a lot today and yesterday. It must be PMS again or something of the sort.

October 28, 1987

I've really got to get myself re-motivated and redirected with my eating habits. I've been slipping into bad fat habits lately and it showed with a four pound gain in two weeks. Ugh! It's time to get all fired up to get that last fifteen pounds off.

November 12, 1987

Weigh in today. My weight is not changed from last week. I was so disappointed, I was sure it would be down. Maybe it was that dinner and cheese cake I ate over at my friend's last night.

November 15, 1987

We had friends over for fresh trout last night. I really overate—cookies, main dish, and homemade strawberry ice-cream.

Here's another set of measurements looking better than the last. Breastfeeding and walking must have been paying off. Somewhere in between the binging I was doing enough starving or walking or breastfeeding or something to keep the weight going down.

December 1, 1987

Bust 35"

Waist 26"

Hip 36"

Thigh 21"

The year 1987 closed with me still fixated on weight, having had some success with losing, but facing another dreaded Christmas season. I continued to see the dietician for weight checks in the New Year.

# The taste of defeat

Once starting on sugar, I seemed to be on a slippery slope that was near impossible to get off. Every Christmas season seemed to fuel the slippery slope and taste of defeat.

> January 6, 1988
>
> My first weigh in since before the holidays—I gained 2¾ pounds. I was actually quite pleased that it wasn't a bigger gain. So here I go again.

The pattern of eating to cope with disappointments, big and small, continued as recorded in the next journal entry.

> January 12, 1988
>
> I finished knitting a sweater for a friend's baby shower. I was disappointed when I got the sweater sewn up and realized I had no zipper for it. I was so discouraged and so upset that I had spent all those hours on it and didn't like it. I made a batch of oatmeal cookies. Joan and I ate the whole bunch. That made me more upset. Then I took the kids out for their sleigh ride. After my walk in the fresh air I felt better and thought that the sweater didn't look so bad after all.
>
> I went to the shower and I overate on the crackers and cheese. Blast it!

January 13, 1988

I paid for my gorging on cookies and cheese: weight up by two pounds. Yipe! I've got to stop this and get on the downward trend again.

January 15, 1988

My goal now for weight is to get down to 125 pounds by April 1st, our fifth anniversary. That is eleven weeks away and that's what I'm going to do. I've got to get remotivated to get these last fourteen pounds off. It's so annoying to gain and have to lose the same pounds over again. I'm going to do it. I'm going to walk that fat off and I'm going to be lean and fit and healthy.

Food was not only a coping mechanism for disappointments, but also a tool for dealing with the anxiety of social situations. When my children were small, their father played in a recreation volleyball league and we frequently went along to be with him on weekend tournaments. Hardly a holiday for me, they proved a bigger stress entertaining two active toddlers in a gymnasium while watching games. But that was the easy part. The hard part was the evening socials where I sat feeling horribly out of place while the team revelled or commiserated about their game plays. Food was the only thing that seemed to want me there or notice me, so my love affair with it continued.

January 17, 1988

I overate yesterday and today—lots of fat stuff—pizza etc. I completely lost control and ate and ate and ate. Ah well, that is now behind me. My dreams are still alive before me.

Last night we had pizza with the volleyball players then went to the hotel and watched TV before going to sleep.

This morning I had a fattening breakfast then sat in the hot tub for a while and came home.

Knowing me, I likely starved between the last entry and the next in preparation for the dreaded weigh in.

### January 20, 1988

Weigh in. I am down to 137 ½ pounds—two pounds lost. That was a good way to start the day.

# Night terrors

The next entry baffled me more. What the hell was I doing working a night shift, caring for small children, and trying to be all things to all people? No wonder I was so stressed and eating myself into oblivion! Sleep deprivation has always flipped me into food binging. I felt that I had to work because I felt that my then husband was not at all interested in supporting a family and I lacked the guts to address the issue. It was too demoralizing to have to ask for grocery money. It was easier to just eat the anxiety away rather than bring up the volatile issue of money.

<u>March 16, 1988</u>

What a dreadful week I've had emotionally. I've felt like a wrung out rag, devoid of any energy or motivation—the self-hate syndrome. I've been telling myself that my period starting today was to blame i.e. PMS. Then I said it was the night shift I worked Sunday. I've felt like a rag since that night shift, like I'm trying to get over jet lag. For two days I've been eating uncontrollably and I feel like a bloated cow. Blast! I've got to get a hold of myself and get out of this downward spin I'm on. I can't stand this any longer. I must get control again and get out of the doldrums of doing nothing.

> March 20, 1988
>
> I'm back in better control of my life now. I started walking again in the early morning. That gives me a great emotional boost for the day.

A few months later I was once again in a bad eating mode. At this time, I was working part time as a nurse, caring for two small children, a large garden, and an acre of raspberries, as well as serving as the president of a church women's auxiliary. Things came to a fat head with this next entry.

> June 13, 1988
>
> I am feeling very stressed and torn lately. I have too many "masters" to serve. Too many voices yelling—hospital, church, family, community, personal needs, house needs. I finally decided something had to go so I quit work. There's no need to have that taking up time too. I just can't cut it. I'm going to fall apart if I keep it all up. Work had to go before church.
>
> I know I'm stressed because I've been overeating on junk food. That's a sure sign that I don't want to face certain things in my life. I'm fasting tomorrow to see if I can't call on some reserve spiritual and emotional strength to turn the tide to a more positive note. Food binging certainly doesn't help. Walking does, but I've not been fitting that in lately either.

I walked and ate my way through another year managing, at least on the surface, to keep life afloat without running away screaming and binging into the woods. Not only did I have too much on my food plate, my life plate was much too large for any rational human. Besides that, I had a husband who took life in even greater gulps than I did—always working 24/7 and adding more to his already over-filled schedule. The more he worked, the more I ate. If that wasn't enough, the plate was about to get even fuller.

# Way too much on my plate

Over a year went by before I again mention dieting and weight in my journal writings. My life plate continued to be filled with my children, family, and church responsibilities. I became pregnant with my third child in the fall of 1988. Once again pregnancy became a food free-for-all. Not only did I have too much on my food plate, I had way too much on my life plate—caring for children, church service, looking after an acre of raspberries, chasing cattle, and trying to maintain a household. I was living life in huge gulps the same way I ate.

The summer of 1989 was by far the fattest and most hectic thus far in my life.

June 22, 1989

I'm very large again with lots of excess weight and am looking forward to shedding it all soon. About two months to go and I'll be unpregnant again. Hooray. I had an ultrasound at five months, which showed a normal single fetus. Alas, the excess weight is me and not an extra baby. Ah well, it came off before so it will come off again.

June 23, 1989

My hands and feet feel tight tonight—must be bloating time again. I'm so big and life is much more difficult when you're fat.

We had a steer get out today. I get winded very quickly chasing cattle. This excess weight is really the pits.

July 10, 1989

I feel like I'm ready to explode. I'm so big, very few clothes fit, and moving from one point to another is becoming increasingly difficult.

I delivered my third child, John Gordon, on August 17, 1989 after travelling most of the day from Calgary, Alberta to home (a six hour drive) after delivering a load of raspberry sales. For two months I had not had a doctor's visit due to the hectic schedule I had looking after a commercial raspberry patch and transporting raspberries to Calgary for sale. No wonder I did not have time to write in my journal until fall set in.

October 25, 1989

The passage of time is such a wonderful thing. I did survive the summer and what a relief it has passed. Raspberry season was a nightmare as usual. I made nine trips to Calgary with berries and they all sold. I bloated terribly with fluid retention, but that all came to an end too when I delivered on August 17th.

I'm not sure what my weight actually climbed to, but it was over 200 pounds. Five days after delivery I weighed 178 pounds and have been dropping steadily since. Four weeks ago I got started on my walking program and am doing four miles in an hour now.

October 30, 1989

I read in the new Reader's Digest an article called "The Paunch Line" about fat distribution and heart disease risk. My shape—pear—is lower risk; however fat on the thighs and hips is almost impossible to get rid of. According to research, the only activity that triggers fat loss from hips and thighs is lactation. I was happy to hear that. I am happily lactating.

I want to be thin and fit.

My lofty aspirations once again take off as I look to the future to being an elite athlete. An Abba song comes to mind: "I have a dream, a fantasy; to help me through reality," or something like that. What is for sure is that I DID need a fantasy to get me through the challenges in my life, the greatest being my inability to advocate for myself and ask for what I needed.

November 2, 1989

I'm back into the great feeling of walking. I started my walking again when Gordon was six weeks old. The first few times were drudgery. I was out of shape and puffing away. Now I feel good again and have been going five weeks.

December 8, 1989

Tonight we went out to the church Christmas party.

I stuffed myself into the green skirt and top that I got on my birthday last year. I felt a bit bulgy in it, but didn't have anything else. I tried my blue jumpsuit, but my husband said I looked worse in it, especially from the rear. I've lost 26 pounds in 3½ months. Another 26 pounds and I'll really look lean. How wonderful that will be!

# As a woman thinketh in her thighs so is she

During the year I continued to read books on positive thinking and visualization. I clipped pictures of thin models from catalogues and placed them at strategic places in my kitchen with notes attached: 'I deserve to weigh 120 pounds.' I was psyching myself up for success with positive self-talk and planting the image in my brain. As 1989 turned into 1990 I was armed and ready to get into the best shape of my life. The following journal entries show my determination and hopeful exercise routine.

January 3, 1990

I am certain that this is the year I'll get my body to the weight of 120 pounds and shape that I imagine myself to be. 1990 is going to be a good year for me. I have a really good feeling. I'm going to be successful in getting my weight to 120 pounds. I deserve to weigh 120 pounds. I know I do.

January 5, 1990

I'm doing the Victoria Principal exercises to tone up my muscles while I'm losing fat.

January 11, 1990

The past few days have been beautiful and sunny. A friend and I have been out walking together every day this week.

The walking, wishing, visualizing, breastfeeding, and eating paid off. By summer I was slim again.

June 5, 1990

I'm glad it's not nine months ago when I had a newborn home and was packing that extra forty plus pounds of fat. My weight is down to 133 pounds and I'm feeling good.

By the time my third child was a year old, I was slim. Slim at last; slim at last; thank God, I was slim at last! Determined to stay slim, I focused on exercise, exercise, and more exercise. I bought size six Land's End jeans. I had arrived! I was slim.

October 2, 1990

Joan and I are taking ballet lessons once a week. I've always wanted to take ballet to feel graceful. I want to get into active "slim" things to keep myself from getting fat again. What a constant eternal battle that is! I'm thin now and I want to stay that way.

Well into winter I record my next food obsession entry. Emotional eating does not end with slimness. With a veterinarian husband workaholic, I had many days, evenings, and nights alone with my three small children. Dark winter days and no TV to boot! What's a foodaholic to do? Eat!

February 4, 1991

We spent the weekend in Spokane and ate too much as usual.

Eating seems to start when I am somewhere between agitation and frustration. Before we hit the Large and Tall store my husband hadn't found anything. He was very irritated and of course that immediately irritates me. Besides having three restless children on hand. We left their dad alone to shop and went on to find snacks, the pet entertainment in such a situation. I suffered today from my excesses of yesterday.

February 10, 1991

Something about Sundays is really depressing to me. After wrestling my children at church I come home to an empty house and felt very lonely. My husband had calls all day. I almost always feel so lonely on Sunday and eat my way through the day. Today was a dark damp dreary day besides.

February 11, 1991

I had a terrible eating binge today. It started with lunch. For some reason I got started eating, then when I went out to drive Joan over to a friend's I saw a bag of cheezies that were left in the car. I ate most of those, and then Marshall and I stopped at the Trading Post. I bought M&M's and two almond joy bars and ate those. Then I ate while I prepared supper, then after supper we bought some ice cream. We ate the whole litre. Now I feel like a stuck pig and rightfully so.

As the dreariness of winter passed, I started biking with my children. A pull-along cart for the baby and bikes for the older ones made the workout a family affair. When the older ones tired out, their bikes were put in the cart along with them and I pulled everyone home, still determined to keep the fat at bay.

<u>March 23, 1991</u>

I am willing to do whatever it takes to have a lean fit body. I am back to regular six mile walks and I'm getting out on my bike as well now that the weather is improving. I can take all my children along so they're a part of it as well.

Just when I had the routine of three children figured out (or at least, fantasized that I did), a new chapter enters my life—baby number four.

# Tour de food begins again

By the fall of 1991 I was pregnant with my fourth child, and yes, I do know what causes it. I AM a nurse you know. Once again I was so relieved to use pregnancy as an excuse to eat without restraint and let it all hang out. If that wasn't enough, that year my then husband decided to open a fitness center that I would manage, so during my pregnancy I took courses on weight training and became a certified weight training instructor.

The gym opened and I was responsible for a certain number of hours running it each day. My stress level escalated, my eating intensified, and my weight increased at a never before seen rate. The stress of being in a gym while gaining weight just made eating worse.

I felt overwhelmed and suffocated by the immense responsibilities placed upon me. All I wanted was to be a mother and homemaker and I found myself caught up in the workaholic habits of my husband. Silenced and sullen, I was too gutless to voice my opinions, so I ate to assuage the anger settling on my thighs.

My journal is uncharacteristically silent for some time on weight issues. I can only surmise that I had given up and decided to throw calories to the wind and eat whatever, whenever, with whomever. I recall nights having take-out pizza (two for one) for my family. While they ate one, I ate the other. The bigger I got, the more I ate.

On June 1, 1992 I gave birth to my fourth child, Alicia Joy. According to memory, I gained more with her than with my other three children (but I still love her).

My next journal entry focusing on weight is after her birth when I was back to the gym to get fit again.

<u>July 28, 1992</u>

I've been working out at the gym regularly since mid-June and I feel better physically. As usual I packed on a lot of excess fat, which I am now working off again. Up down, up down. Hopefully, this will be my last fat time.

As I struggled with the care of four children, myself, a marriage, and managing a fitness center (something I hated), I often felt overwhelmed with everything there was to do. Not much is written during that year about anything in my life. One journal line amidst others, written on October 12, 1992, kind of sums it up. "We've had a very stressful and unpleasant year."

## Binged there, ate that

My memory is that I had a number of diet gimmicks that I tried during this time. I learned about brain gym from a friend and off we went to the States (breastfeeding baby in tow) to attend a workshop. Brain gym was going to be the key to getting my brain fit and fixed on health and weight loss rather than holding on to my weight. I wish I had the money and time back that I spent on it!

After brain gym I bought an ear piece that promised acupressure points that would decrease my appetite. It lasted about a month then I couldn't be bothered readjusting it and taking care of it. The butt line is that I really didn't think it would work and it didn't. Besides, food addiction is not about physical appetite. I rarely ate for hunger. I ate for lust and hate and fear and loneliness and guilt and remorse and jealousy and anger and frustration and whatever other emotions I couldn't seem to manage.

Then there were the subliminal tapes I listened to every night that were supposed to reprogram my bad brain habits or whatever was making me eat and eat and eat. I don't remember how long I lasted at this strategy, but it too came to an end.

With that or despite all that I still managed to once again get rid of my excess weight. Breastfeeding seemed to be magic for me. Either that or it was just my belief that it was magic for me. I also continued my daily walking, something that does more for my emotional health than any other thing I do in my day. By the time my fourth and last baby was a year old, I was back down to a weight somewhere in the 135 pound range and feeling again that I had arrived.

My hectic life must have influenced the lack of journaling in 1993. Only a few entries are recorded that year, none of them discussing my weight or dieting. Still breastfeeding and still walking likely kept my weight in a range comfortable for me. In the spring of 1994 I wrote about the wonderful feelings associated with walking.

April 4, 1994

There are two things I really enjoy doing: one is walking, the other is eating. Few things give me a happier, more optimistic outlook than brisk walking for several miles. I love the wonderful tingling feeling my every cell experiences. It's like every little atom in my body is euphoric and celebrating life. I love the alive feeling and even my biggest problems don't bother me if I've started the day out with a good long walk. This morning I got in about ten miles and I feel ready to conquer the world. I'm so elated. My body loves exercise and I love to sit down to a wonderful banquet too and enjoy each course to the fullest. Maybe even have an extra dish of ice-cream which is my favorite dessert.

The euphoria of weight management through walking and breastfeeding eventually came to an end. Alas, I could not breastfeed forever. That sucked!

# The binge hour

It seemed that as soon as my daughter was weaned, somewhere around age two, I started to gain weight and, despite my determination to never be fat again, less than a year later I found myself again battling with fat. Around this time I bought a book called the *Carbohydrate Addict's Diet*. I was so excited with the thought that I could binge for one hour a day and lose weight. So binge I did. I planned great feasts with scrumptious desserts. I lined up all the food I wanted to eat and got it ready for the binge hour, and then I ate. It was worth your life to get between me and my food for that one hour. I enlisted a plump friend (taking her down with me, in weight I mean) and she jumped on the hourly binge bandwagon with me and for a while we both lost weight, but inevitably it stopped working. The pounds came back faster than before and left me with a bigger butt and appetite for desserts and junk food than I had ever before had.

Another failed attempt at weight management left me once again despairingly introspective about myself. The desperation and despair mingled with my ever (almost ever) present humor is clear in this next entry.

<u>March 29, 1995</u>

I've spent a lot of thought wallowing in despair at my size. I wonder why it is such an obsession and a torment to me. I've been major walking for almost three months now and the size of my lower body, meaning my hips, butt, and thighs, has not changed noticeably. By major walking, I mean like 8-11 miles a day averaging 5-6 days a week. Like, I mean I've been walking – race walking. But why is this such a burden to me? I want to just let it all go and never again labor over a fat gram or calorie or size or what to eat. I want to be free just to live and enjoy, to never feel hunger or guilt because I've eaten ice-cream or whatever the food of the day is. Maybe if I write it all out I'll get it off my chest and out of my mind. I just can't take the burden anymore. I enjoy walking; I just don't understand how I could not decrease my fat by the amount of exercise I've been getting. I'm sure that everyone is tired of hearing me pontificate on weight and diet and size and fat grams and to eat wheat or not to eat wheat, to drink hot water or cold water... I'm tired of hearing myself. I think I'm suffering from information overload and if I just relaxed and lived, it might all go away.

My husband says I'm too focused on it. He also says if I hadn't had such intense major eating the month of December I wouldn't be suffering now. Probably right, but the more he gives me advice on not eating, the more I eat. I really did outdo myself baking and eating this Christmas. So he says none of us need all that baking and such even if it is Christmas. So I swore with an oath as did Chief Joseph, "I will bake no more forever," I said. That's easy right now because my oven is shot and no one seems in a hurry to repair it. But already I feel beckoned by a rhubarb pie (I happened to have seen frozen rhubarb in my freezer today). I'm not even a baker really, I'm just an eater, but I'm an athlete too. I really am. I get hours of race walking in each week. So is it going to take a stick of dynamite to blow my butt and thighs off or should I just relax and forget about it? That's what I'd really like to do, but I'm afraid of getting fatter. I don't even know why I have such a fat phobia or why I'm so tormented by it. Why me?

One thing for sure is that we always get what we deserve either in this life or in the life to come.

So why then do I deserve torment over my size? My husband says in my last incarnation I must have been skinny and made fun of fat people. I'm not into reincarnation, but if I ever did, I'm very sorry, and I repent now speedily and timely to rid myself of my struggle. It's so senseless to feel guilty for eating. Like, look at all the scum bags in this world—rapists, murderers, thieves, crooks, politicians etc. – so why would I feel guilty for eating? Or for being size twelve or for having cellulite on my thighs? Get a life! I have to go now because it's time to get my children up for school.

God bless my precious children. They kept me going through all my emotional and physical ups and downs.

## Built like a house

In the 90s I read a book about lightening up your life to lighten up your body. All I had to do was to look at my surroundings in my home and see a similarity between the condition of my body and the condition of my house. Sure enough, there I was, looking just like my house. I stuffed all my clutter into the basement to hide it from view and there I was also with all my excess weight settled on my metaphorical basement—my butt and thighs. I sucked as much at keeping my house as I did at keeping my weight.

I went on the proverbial house tornado routine, cleaning and purging and tossing stuff out. I emptied the basement and decluttered myself damn near into a coma, but there I was, still big in my body basement. Another fat theory shot all to hell. No matter what my housekeeping was like, my fat keeping remained unchanged.

Keeping my children kept me going no matter what and that is what happened. Fat or thin, slob or clean, I was motivated by love to carry on and care for my precious children. Two months after that last weight misery entry, I revisited goals for weight loss. My fortieth birthday was rapidly approaching. It was time to get serious about my weight. I so much did not want to be fair, fat, and forty.

May 22, 1995

Twenty weeks from this day I will be forty years old. What I really want for my fortieth birthday is to be lean, to be really lean, and free of unsightly bulges. I'm going off sugar and junk from now 'til then—focus on super health. I'm considering getting a private weight loss counsellor. I know one who's also a nurse and I may call to get her help through the next few months.

I walked the ten kilometre Blossom Run in one hour and fifteen minutes. I was the only walker, so I was way behind everyone, but I still had pretty good time for me. I could do it faster, especially if I wasn't packing so much fat.

Enter the period of private diet counseling—a new venture for me. I worked with a nurse who lost weight eating a diabetic diet and then started a private diet counseling business in her home. It seemed to be what I needed for a time. I trusted her because I had known her when she was overweight, so I felt that she could understand my weight plight.

July 5, 1995

On May 31st I went to see my nurse colleague re: diet counseling and have been seeing her weekly for weighing. I finally decided that I needed outside help and I'm glad I did, although it was a disheartening shock to be weighed and admit I had gained so much. My weight then was 170 pounds. I've lost ten pounds since and am not terribly uncomfortable with her eating plan which follows a diabetic diet.

I've been doing major cycling around the valley this past month. I started cycling when blisters stopped me from walking. My new walking shoes proved to be the shoes from hell. My feet are near healed again, I even did some five mile walks in socks. I should design a walking sock. It's much lighter and easier than shoes.

My biggest bike ride was on Canada Day. I got up early and biked all the way to Wynndel on the lower road then back on the upper road. That was a hard 3½ hour ride. By the time I got home I was starving and my legs were trembling. But I love the feel of being fit.

August 9, 1995

Since June 1st I've now dropped sixteen pounds. This week's weigh in was disappointing. I had such a good week and was expecting to have lost maybe three pounds but the scale stayed the same. I was so disappointed because I had exercised major amounts and stuck to low fat food. We went on a holiday, two nights at Champion Lakes then three nights at Christina Lake. I walked every day and swam and treaded water and hiked. I felt so slim until I weighed in. Then I wanted to sit down and believe it's a hopeless cause. But I remind myself that I'm sixteen pounds less than I was 2½ months ago, so there's no reason to weep. Maybe next week will show a drop.

My weight problems did not seem to be a lack of exercise. Exercise was something I very much enjoyed, I just couldn't seem to manage the intake of food, or maybe it was my emotions that I couldn't manage. As I recall I had lost a fair amount of weight by my fortieth birthday. Once the day was over, it was back to eating as usual. Getting through the fall and Christmas of 1995 left me fat again and sick and tired of dieting. A new era dawned, an epiphany of sorts: no more dieting.

## From where the cellulite now sets, I will diet no more forever

As 1996 came upon me I was totally exhausted with the whole weight obsession. I was spent. I was worn out with the ups and downs of dieting and weight. I was so done! It was time to let it go, but not quite let it go, just let it go in bits and pieces. How could I start a new year without some form of dieting?

January 17, 1996

This year I vowed not to sweat about my weight (emotionally, I mean). One thing only I gave up and that was sugar. So by the time I got through the holiday eating it was January 8th that I started no sugar. So far, over a week now, I've been sugar free, no artificial sweeteners either, except in very minute amounts.

The first few days weren't bad, then I had a lingering headache for 4-5 days. I actually do feel much better and don't seem to crave food so much. I feel more balanced like I don't need to stuff myself then starve, then stuff, then starve. You know the old stuff and starve routine where it's either feast or famine but never balanced, like I'm teetering on the brink of something.

Not sweating over my weight didn't seem to help either. I continued to gain through the winter, trying desperately not to diet. It turned out to be harder to not diet than to diet. Now what? The fat war continued and with it the pathetic and perplexing obsession.

March 5, 1996

I'm sure spring really is close, but this snow setback makes it look grim. It's like gaining back the ten pounds you just lost. I know my life revolves around weight but I am trying desperately to not diet and to be "normal", whatever that is. What is so appealing about munching and crunching and swallowing? What is so wonderful about that hand to mouth motion of eating? Why doesn't broccoli taste like chocolate? Why isn't cauliflower addictive? It doesn't seem fair that something as gross as spinach is so packed with nutrients and something as yummy as rocky-road ice-cream is so bad for you. I wish taste buds craved kale and cabbage. Trying to keep my weight from going up is like trying to contain an oil slick. I feel like I constantly work just to keep from spreading too fast, like it's a major effort to keep my head above water or to keep my thighs and butt the same size as my last purchased pair of jeans. Is there any hope for me?

I love to move. That's not the problem. I really get a lot of exercise. I like to walk, cycle, do weights etc. In fact, if I had no other responsibility in life I'd spend all my time exercising.

I just want to be lean, but it seems to elude me. I might as well wish for a million dollars it seems. To dream the impossible dream!

## March 6, 1996

A friend thinks I should join Weight Watchers with her. There's a session of ten weeks starting again soon. It's on my mind. One of my nurse colleagues went to Weight Watchers two years ago and lost thirty pounds and looks wonderful. She's got her life-time membership now and goes monthly. She looks so trim. I'm jealous. Maybe I need a lifetime something or other to take care of my weight.

## March 30, 1996

For the past two weeks I've been coughing and spitting and snorting. I was getting very exhausted from coughing 'til I vomited a couple times. I finally started taking some Amoxicillin that my husband brought home for the dog.

The lack of appetite was a plus. I shrunk enough fat away to comfortably get into my jeans again. One must always look at the positive side.

The proverbial cup half full and plate fully full continued.

# Big sugar

The short-lived illness and weight loss gave way to more obsessing about food and size. With each passing month the mystery and misery with the problem intensified.

<u>June 10, 1996</u>

Lately, all I want to do is sleep and eat and I'm wondering why I constantly have this same old problem cropping up again and again and again. What do I need to resolve? Is it a physical addiction to food? Is it an emotional problem? Or just laziness? I want to somehow resolve this problem. I can't get interested in losing weight anymore because I believe it will only come back again. This has been going on for over twenty years, my quest for thinness. Here I am still fat, none of my jeans fitting, and wishing I could go to a dry out center for food drunks.

My no sugar vow lasted until Joan's birthday. How can I get through birthdays and holidays and summer and parenting without treats? What's a mother to do? I keep telling myself I'm just going to relax and accept myself fat, but the truth is I really hate being fat. I hate feeling my thighs rub together and rolls hanging over my pants waist, and I really hate seeing double chins on my face. Someday I wish I had to dig ditches all day so I had no food around me. Should I change the subject or should I continue to hash this out page after page after page? The truth is that I don't like myself when I'm eating uncontrollably, especially when I get eating sugar and junk food (who pigs out on kale?). I start really envying people who are perennially thin. Why wasn't I born with that rapid BMR that they all boast about?

I don't even want to go out walking or cycling anymore. I feel like "what's the use?" It doesn't seem to work anymore. Even my children are asking, "Mom, why don't you ever lose weight with all the walking you do?" I don't know.

Losing weight is like cleaning. Why clean up? It's just going to get messy again. Why lose weight? It's just going to come back again. I might as well accept life as a fat person, buy big clothes, and carry on.

The truth is I really want to be thin, like really lean, no bulges, no cellulite, no love handles, just very lean. I really want to be lean. I really want to be lean. I really want to be lean.

9:25 p.m. I still really want to be lean. I successfully rested my system today with only water.

I still really want to be lean. If I were lean, my children wouldn't fight, my house wouldn't get messy, my husband wouldn't be a workaholic, and I probably wouldn't have freckles either. I'd probably be five inches taller too.

# Hungry games

My mind games and thigh games and stomach and extreme eating and fasting games continued.

June 11, 1996

I still really want to be lean and I'm going to keep reminding myself of this, the same that I want to be a good person. I feel much brighter and happier this morning having fasted for 24 hours than I did yesterday waking with a food hangover. I honestly feel happier and more energetic without eating. I had a green apple this morning and a tablespoon of linseed oil (that's my latest fad – I read it would help balance your metabolism and help lose weight). "Whatever it takes."

June 12, 1996

5:45 a.m. I just came in from a four mile walk/jog combo and I'm feeling quite well. I still really want to be thin. I mean like really lean—no bulges, no bumps or lumps, no extra chins. I even want lean toes.

I feel good this morning even though I had ice-cream cake for a family birthday last night.

June 13, 1996

I got out for another good walk/jog this morning. I still really want to be lean. I'm trying life without sugar again. A friend loaned me a book on hypoglycemia. She's been sugar and refined flour free for about seven years because of her reaction to sugar. I think I have similar problems with sugar—the headaches, irritability, sleepiness, and depression. I definitely feel happier when I don't eat it. I really have to keep reminding myself of that.

I really want to be thin—like really want to be thin.

June 14, 1996

I got a call from the bicycle shop that my pull cart was fixed and ready to go. So I biked into town (eight miles) with Alicia on the bike seat then picked up the cart and biked home.

June 15, 1996

I really enjoyed yesterday spending most of the day physically moving. I could quite happily bike, walk, rollerblade, swim, climb, or hike all day with just meal breaks and maybe one afternoon nap and stretching time. Perhaps that lifestyle would make me thin. I've been wishing and praying for eternal thinness to happen no matter what I eat or drink. As I was out biking across the wishing bridge the thought occurred that what I should plead for is to love a healthy lifestyle so much that the sugar and overindulgent lifestyle would only repulse me.

My jean shorts seemed tighter this morning than last time I wore them and that makes me angry. I still really want to be thin, to be light and quick.

June 18, 1996

I'm feeling irritable, probably from the chocolate brownies I ate yesterday. Don't ask me why I made brownies. I don't think I've ever made brownies before. I feel like having a good cry.

# Angry dieter

I still get angry and cravings for food when I look at these entries in which I suffered through the agony of night shifts, dreading every minute of them, and wanting to be home with my family full-time. If the person I am now could go back to that time, I would assert myself and make my needs and desires known. Above all, I would NOT have continued to work while having children at home. I know, I know! Hindsight is always better than diet sight.

<u>July 17, 1996</u>

I bought a new diet book yesterday—my favorite pastime. This one is the rotation diet and I'm going to start it on Friday after my night shifts are over. Tune in, the book promises a loss of ⅔ pounds per day and maybe one pound a day for strict adherence to the plan. I wouldn't mind losing twenty pounds in a month take a short break then lose another twenty pounds. Who wouldn't want those results? So here's to another diet.

My goal is to not talk about this diet to anyone and to just quietly do it. Do you think that's possible?

<u>July 20, 1996</u>

Day two of the rotation diet and all's well. I feel slimmer already.

<u>July 21, 1996</u>

Day three of the rotation diet and all's well.

I know I can lose this fat. I know I can. I know I can be slim. It is possible. I keep thinking of others who've done it and that gives me hope.

<u>July 25, 1996</u>

I'm doing well on day seven. I've got through these seven days very well with very little more than the allowed calories. I know I can do it. I'm feeling very motivated and my desire is strong. I really want to be thin. No bumps, no bulges, no excess curves and lumps—just a clean straight lean line. Is that too much to ask?

Monday, I worked in ER. I walked to work, a two hour walk, but felt great. I met up with a former heart patient out walking and heard his motivating story of lifestyle change and loss of 94 pounds. It was an uplifting walk.

On Tuesday I biked the loop to town and back, another good two hour workout. Yesterday I walked four miles.

<u>July 28, 1996</u>

This morning I went for an hour walk with Marshall biking along.

### August 1, 1996

I've had two weeks of surviving my diet. This has been the hardest day for some reason. Perhaps because I'm just feeling restless, irritable, and wishing I could have at least a full day of undisturbed solitude.

### August 8, 1996

This is the 21st day of my diet and I'm feeling good. I'm going to keep this up. It feels so much better to be in control, to be exercising each day, and knowing my body is not overburdened with excess food, especially junk food. It's too bad I didn't weigh myself three weeks ago so I'd know how successful this eating plan is. Ah well, I did weigh myself a week ago in ER, so I'll check again tomorrow when I work. At least I'll know what this past week did. I've had loads of walking and biking, so I'm hoping for a significant loss.

The rotation diet was a ridiculously low calorie diet, near starvation, going from five to eight hundred calories per day. It was certainly predictable that I wouldn't keep that going for long. During a motor home holiday on my own with four children (ages four, seven, nine, and eleven) to Saskatchewan (a two day drive one way) my rotation diet rotated right out of my life and into the prairie sunset and I turned it into the bloatation diet instead. My dieting journal was silent for a few months, resurfacing on that fattest of fat holidays—Halloween.

### October 31, 1996

Boy! Another diet shot all to hell. Actually it went out with my holiday to Prince Albert in the last two weeks of August.

It's Halloween and I know I'm going to eat myself into a frenzy and I haven't solved any of my fat problems. Another year rolls to a close and I'm still my usual rolly polly self. Ah well, bring on the chocolate!

Another year of dieting failure came to a close leaving me still fat, so what was the point of the rotation diet misery in between?

## My magic fat free kingdom

I started 1997 with a family vacation to Mexico, travelling via motor home. I remember being so disgusted with myself that I had no clothes to wear because nothing fit. I had to buy a few outfits of fat clothes that I could wear for the holiday. Throwing diet and fat to the wind (well, not really, I still fantasized about the coming year and what it might do for my weight loss dreams), I determined to enjoy the vacation with my family—Disneyland and all.

My strategy for 1997 was to focus more on exercise than on diet. I remember firmly proclaiming that the fat war was over. The fat had won and I no longer cared. I pronounced my defeat to fat with the same zeal and conviction that I had previously pronounced all my commitments to weight loss diets. But, like all my previous diet proclamations, this one too proved to be vain.

The journal entries for 1997 begin while travelling in a motor home with my family on the way home from a holiday to Mazatlan. The vacation gave me time to dream again of being an athlete. I just kept believing that if I could just exercise enough, I could eat whatever and whenever I wanted. Ah, if life were like that, I wouldn't have needed Visa to buy the magic running shoes I bought.

### January 26, 1997 Tucson, Arizona

I got a book on running (my next fad). I got a pair of Nike Triax Max Air running shoes. I hope they'll turn me into a runner.

### January 30, 1997

I'm bored with travelling and chowing down on Oreos (reduced fat, of course) and fat-free fig bars. Who am I trying to kid? I ate too much pizza for supper—definitely not reduced or fat free. I swam for a while with my children then had a good long look at myself nude in the motel room. Yikes! I hope running will help my body. I know what I want. I want to be ultra-lean and muscular. I want to look like a distance runner.

### January 31, 1997

I'm up early, dressed, and ready to go home. Happy, happy day! I'll get to sleep in my own bed tonight. I'll get back into a healthy routine and spring is not far off.

I've eaten ten fig bars while writing this. It should be good for the bowels.

Winters and weight gain continued to go hand in hand and mouth in mouth from thigh to spreading thigh. I'm not sure why I didn't just call a friend or sister and commiserate rather than isolate myself and eat. That's another of my life's personal mysteries.

### February 5, 1997

I have a sore throat and a bad case of post-holiday blues. I just read in *Prevention* about a 62 year old woman who had at 55 lost thirty pounds and then started exercising and competing in triathlon biking. Hmm, I wonder if that could happen to me.

February 15, 1997

I'm just lying in bed thinking of spring and getting out walking again and getting slim and wondering if it's at all possible anymore. I know I'd feel better if I could just get walking regularly again. I really do want to be fit. I want to be a runner but I want to enjoy running.

Predictably the passage of winter to spring brought with it an increase in mood and motivation. Something about the arrival of spring in the great white north awakens the optimistic spirit again. Spring came again to my winter laden moods.

April 2, 1997

I got out walking early morning the past two days. I feel a lot better already, but tonight I feel bloated and heavy even though I've not overindulged.

May 11, 1997

Gorgeous day. I've kept up my daily exercise since April 1st. I've missed only two days since then. My running has advanced very quickly. Yesterday I ran eleven kilometres from here to the Pizza Factory, and then I walked up the hill to the hospital and worked a twelve hour day shift.

June 7, 1997

I am still keeping up with running, some days walking. I'm feeling fit. I still have a load of fat to lose, but I'm feeling good.

## June 12, 1997

I bought some chocolate mint cookies and had a good pig out. That's part of my life and doing it less and less frequently is now my goal. To say I will never overeat again is to become perfect overnight. Now I'm content to say I will get exercise most days and eat sensibly most days and that's okay.

Running lasted for a while then predictably I abandoned that too. I never liked running so how was I ever going to maintain that regime for a lifetime?

When my youngest child started kindergarten in 1997 I was convinced that now I would have the time to exercise enough that I would no longer be fat. Finally I could eat anything I wanted and have the time to work it off, or so I thought. I used her three hour time at school each day for walking. I walked and I walked and I walked. Yet I was still chubby after all those walks!

# Just get a life!

In the fall of 1997, a strange dream that I had terminal cancer seemed to wake me from my self-pity and remind me that there are worse things in life than being fat.

The effect of that dream seemed to stop my self-pity about weight for a time and I decided to just get a life. I proclaimed self-acceptance, swore myself off dieting, and allowed the fat to win. Still continuing to walk, I decided to buy the clothes I wanted in the size I was and quit waiting for some magical size before buying decent clothes.

December 4, 1997

> Beautiful weather still. Sunny afternoon yesterday and I had a wonderful walk. It's so exhilarating to go out walking outside. I love the way it makes me feel—the movement, the fresh air, the sights and sounds.
>
> Last week I got myself a gorgeous dark olive wool crepe suit from the Talbots catalogue. Expensive, but gorgeous. I felt so elegant and sophisticated wearing it to church on Sunday. It doesn't matter so much that it's a size fourteen. I still felt elegant, sleek, and beautiful.

I closed out the year feeling okay with myself, fit but not slim. It seemed to be over. I could just live and be at peace with my size. The new year, 1998 started with a family vacation to Cuba.

My first journal entries for 1998 affirm my new-found self-acceptance, planning for fitness goals rather than weight goals.

January 3, 1998

I've got a supply of good books from the church book store in Calgary and a pile of health and fitness magazines to read on the beach. I'll come back all renewed and motivated for improvement. I feel much better than I did a year ago. I've had a good year with exercise, lots of running and walking. I feel fit and strong, not thin, but fit and strong and for now, that's good enough.

January 19, 1998

I want to thoughtfully come up with some good goals for 1998, a.k.a. New Year's resolutions. Now might be a good time to do that. Now for some resolutions:

1. Train for a marathon (I'm afraid to say run a marathon). Why?

By the time spring came, the monster had returned and I was again obsessing about my size.

April 4, 1998

I'm trying to determine what I really want in life aside from wanting to be thin. I looked at myself front and backwards in the mirror. Ouch! The mirror must be at fault.

Perhaps more accurately, what I wanted is to like myself at any size, but that seemed not to be possible then or now. Something about excess weight is just not consistent with feeling good about myself.

# Hawaii Fat-O

Somewhere in the spring of 1998 I made the impulsive decision to move to Hawaii for a year. I am not sure exactly why I did this, except that my journal entries talk about getting out of a familiar rut and getting my children out of their comfortable ruts to see another side of the world. Likely I thought that I would be a different person in a different place and maybe that's what I was searching for or running from or hoping for. My then husband sold his veterinarian practice and wanted to spend time writing a book. Hawaii seemed like a good place to do this, although this was not his plan but mine.

Being a registered nurse, it was fairly easy to secure work and a work permit in Hawaii. So I packed up my children and headed for Hawaii with my husband planning to follow later. As I struggled into life in Hawaii, I make this observation in my journal, still hoping after all these years.

<u>September 20, 1998</u>

I was writing in my journal out on the front step one day last week when an elderly neighbor stopped by to chat. She said that she quit writing in her journal twenty years ago when she realized that all her entries were the same. It sounds like a large part of my life has been hashing over the same weight obsession year after year after year. Secretly I'm hoping that this year in Hawaii might help resolve that somehow.

The change in location provided me with some changes in diet strategies and new people to meet and listen to. The Hawaii workplace was filled with women discussing weight and diet just as my Creston workplace had been. The stress of the move and the grief of homesickness and loneliness initially decreased my appetite. This was a totally new phenomenon to me—I lost my appetite and started to gradually decrease in weight without thinking about it. Typically my mood went up as my weight went down.

October 8, 1998

A nurse I work with tells me papaya is the greatest cleanser for the digestive system. Read, weight loss! So now I eat a couple papayas every day.

October 12, 1998

Am I trying to escape myself, only to find that everywhere I go, there I am still? Maybe I was hoping I would be someone different if I lived in a different place. I'm not sure who I wanted to be except a slim person.

November 24, 1998

Yesterday Joan and I had a wonderful all-day shopping spree in Honolulu. I was excited to fit into size ten pants again. I have lost weight here. The black pants I wore here are much too big now.

<u>December 6, 1998</u>

Marshall and I weighed ourselves for 25¢ on a scale at the Windward mall. He weighs 110 pounds and I weigh 153 pounds, which is twelve pounds less than when we moved here. Yippee skipee.

After the initial stress and culture shock of moving to Hawaii was over, my appetite returned. Alas, I was me again. Damn it!

<u>December 20, 1998</u>

We went to a Christmas open house at the neighbors' down the street. It was a pleasant evening. I ate too much junk food as usual.

Predictably Christmas was an eating orgy. Living in Hawaii did not change this bad habit. I ended the year panicked about the return of the food monster, still spending inordinate amounts of time exercising obsessively to counteract eating obsessively.

For most of my months in Hawaii I couldn't wait to get back to the security of Creston and home. I worked a permanent night job. They were usually very quiet nights, so I had a variety of activities to keep me going during the night—reading books, eating, planning diets, writing outlines for books. My journal entries are much like previous ones—exercising, planning weight loss, obsessing about size. My life did include other things; however this is the focus for this book.

<u>January 4, 1999</u>

I went for a long uphill walk to the town reservoir then went on a 2½ hour bike ride to Sunset Beach and back. My legs are sore.

If I had not recorded the plans for a book like this in my journal of 1999, I would not have remembered having this book plan so long ago. I wish I still had the outline I refer to in this entry.

January 11, 1999

I worked last night and wrote out an outline for a book: All My Sizes, a Chronology of Life's Ups and Downs.

I heard on the radio that fidgeting keeps people thin. I am now a confessed fidgeter.

January 29, 1999

I am sitting out in the sun trying to motivate myself to eat better. I'm on a sugar binge this week. I am still walking everyday but feeling icky with too much junk food flowing through my veins. I wonder why that is? All I really want to accomplish by being away this year is to lose all my excess fat and go home slim, and to increase my spirituality with temple attendance. The temple attendance seems easier than the appetite control. Night shift is particularly bad with tempting me to eat to pass the boredom and to stay awake. I can't seem to run away from the problem, which is me.

February 1, 1999

Idea: questions to ask God:

Why are my thighs so big when I walk so much? Why does my body like to cling to its fat? I could whine a lot about my weight, but being here around so many obese women has made me appreciate my own body. I'm small compared to the average woman here.

I'm not sure what happens to flip me from binging to dieting to moderation and back again. I only know that something changes. The New Atkins diet was being tried and talked about in my workplace so I jumped on this diet wagon for some time and experienced the usual initial success that comes from trying a new diet toy.

February 7, 1999

I am feeling better this week because I've been eating less and eating more nutritiously, so I don't feel fat anymore, or worse, feel out of control. That's the feeling I really don't like.

February 16, 1999

Kahuku hospital
Things to be grateful for:
My weight is improving, as in I'm looking better than a month ago.
My uniform is too big now
My thighs are smaller

February 23, 1999

I tried on a straight skirt in Sears. Size ten fit me. Yippee!

The stress of night shift takes its toll once again and wreaks havoc with my eating patterns as these next entries show.

March 6, 1999

I am feeling night shift hangover like I don't want to do anything so I'm watching the Fox news channel.

LATER: I had a bad eating fury. I went to the store for nacho chips and scarfed them down with salsa. Then my husband got some ice-cream and I scarfed that down too.

Night shift really is the pits. Here I am now, wide awake when everyone else has gone to bed and I just have this one night shift off so I'm eating ice-cream and all I want to do is eat.

March 11, 1999

I'm watching Barney with Alicia. I just scarfed down some ice-cream.

March 26, 1999

I took Alicia and Gordon to a dumb cartoon movie at the theater, *Doug's 1st Movie*. I dozed through it.

I ate too much: a Snicker's bar, some licorice, popcorn, and Sprite. It was boring. What else could I do but eat?

It was time for another bout of Atkins's to make up for the bout of binge eating.

May 2, 1999

I've been doing the Atkins diet for about a month—except for one day I had cake and ice-cream at the neighbor's birthday party. Except for being constipated I don't feel bad. I'm waiting for a day shift to weigh myself at work first thing in the morning.

May 3, 1999

Today I drove to Kaneohe and snooped around the mall. I wanted to get some Atkins protein bars at the health store. I enjoyed being at the mall alone to browse. I tried on some clothes at Sears and bought a casual cotton skirt size eight. I've been trying the same style skirt on for several months. In January the size twelve fit, now the eight fits. I was so happy.

May 25, 1999

I got a measuring tape and measured myself: chest 35"-waist 28"-hips 38"-and thighs 21". Not bad.

Success was short lived. As the diet stopped working, I gave up and started eating again. Food, always, food to soothe my frayed and disappointed nerves.

June 6, 1999

I'm eating like there's not another meal coming. I am totally out of control. I'd like to stay with the Atkins eating but it's not making me lose weight. I haven't lost an ounce in over a month with it. Depressing!

July 12, 1999

I am feeling bloated and full from an ice-cream and chips binge. I don't know why I've got this blues mood. I'm tired of feeling in a temporary setting. I'm ready to be in my own home with my own stuff and carry on for the future.

It seems that I always wanted to be somewhere else, someone else, and some other size. Even when I got to a lean size, I couldn't seem to stay there. My year in paradise ended with me being thin and excited to return to the security of home in the beautiful Creston valley. Certainly I could leave that fat behind in a foreign country without a passport and it wouldn't find me again.

# The real elephant in the room

We left Hawaii and moved back to our home in Creston in August 1999. I was slim when I returned home and relished the numerous compliments on my slimmed down body. Happy as I was to be back in my old home, it wasn't long before the old food habits once again haunted me. Despite getting great amounts of exercise as these journal entries indicate, I started to steadily gain weight.

During this time I also continued working shift work while organizing the busy lives of four active children now ranging in age from seven to fourteen years old. While my children were at school I spent huge blocks of time getting exercise, hoping that the exercise alone would keep my body at the lean level I had managed to get to in Hawaii.

Despite such a high level of exercise and fitness, my slim body quickly faded behind mounting weight gain and with it mounting frustration and despair.

October 12, 1999

Help me! Help me! I'm angry. I'm frustrated. I'm depressed. My pants are all too tight again. I want to cry. I want to scream! I want to eat! Why? Why? Why? I ask. Why can't I stay one size? Why am I spreading again? I can't take this anymore. What's the matter with me?! Help!

By the close of 1999 I had gained over thirty pounds and no longer fit into any of the lovely clothes I had purchased in Hawaii as a slim size eight. The tormenting guilt and shame that go with such a cycle is not even describable. It's hard to go from steady compliments on weight loss to silent stares, knowing that what is being said is not being said to my face. It gives a whole new meaning to the proverbial elephant in the room. Why was I fat again? Why could I not get it? Why would I eat my slim body fat again? What was wrong with me? Where had I gone? I wanted to hide out and eat and dream of that magical Promised Land flowing with size eight clothes, cellulite-free thighs, and sizzling gluts that never spread. With pizza in one hand and a pen in the other, I set out to map, once again, my course to this land of freedom from fat.

# The harder I diet, the fatter I get

What could be more inspiring to a diet addict than the eve of a new millennium? There I sat, having recently gained back thirty pounds of hard-lost fat, still hopeful after all these diet flops. I was as much an optimist addict as I was a food and diet addict.

December 30, 1999

It's time once again for New Year's resolutions. Most of the fun is in the writing and thinking and dreaming of goals to come. I'm sitting by the fire thinking. Actually, I've been pondering year 2000 goals for some time.

1. *eat 10% fat only for the year.*
2. *not weigh myself—not even once for the whole year*
3. *do not mention diet, weight, or fat at all for one year.*

With a New Year, a new decade, and a new millennium dawning, I was certain that this would be the year for me to conquer my food monster. The lofty goals set on the last day of the year were quickly abandoned within a short time as this journal entry shows.

January 10, 2000

I blew this one, meaning number three above.

The misery of night shift prompted me to return to school by distance to get a degree which would expand my options as a professional (unfortunately it expanded my butt as well). My first course was a writing course, which required that I write a *how to* essay. As I pondered about what I am really good at and could write a *how to* essay on, there was no denying I was really good at gaining weight. That essay, written in 2000, is a perfect insert for my book on weight obsession.

*One thing all my diets have taught me is how to gain weight, so if there's anyone out there wanting to gain weight read on. First, go on a diet. Yes, you heard me correctly—go on a diet. It matters not which one you choose, just grab one and fly with it. Look at me, I've tried them all and do you see me having trouble gaining weight? See what I mean? The diets, they all work equally well, the Atkins old or new, the grapefruit, the fit for life, the weight watchers, the weigh down, pray down, lay down and cry diet (I made that one up and I've used it many times—it's very effective). Don't forget to try the south beach, north beach, the no beach, and zone and clone diets. When you're done with those go on to the drastic measures of fasting and starving and concentration camp style eating (these are also great for the budget). The key for this first step in weight gain is to choose the diet.*

*Step two is to announce to everyone you know that you are going on a diet. Tell your family, your friends, your colleagues, pets, plants, and pastor (minister, rabbi, bishop, guru, reverend etc.). It may also be advisable to put an announcement in the local paper – something to let the community at large know of your intent. This is most effectively done around the beginning of the year. Step two ensures that everyone you know will be on the lookout for your dietary habits as well as watching how your clothes fit or do not fit.*

*The next step occurs as soon as you lose enough pounds to go down a size in clothes. It involves throwing out all your large clothes. This is to show your commitment that you are no longer going to be the current size and will look forward to the shopping spree for your new sized body. The method of disposing of the clothes is irrelevant to your overall success. The key here is to just get them out of the house and your life. Some suggestions may be to give the clothes to the local clothing bank, to your church, to sell them at a garage, or to burn them on main street with your bra or feed them to your mother's goats. Just remove them from your plane of vision and from your psyche, for you are now going to be a new smaller size forever!*

*After you have accomplished the above steps, sit back, relax, and watch the weight pile on. I can't tell you how this phenomenon happens, it just does and it may happen within just weeks of starting the diet. The rationale for such success is found in both the physiological and psychological realms of mumbo jumbo, aka behavioral theories. Theory one asserts that after about three weeks (for some it's just three days!) of rigidly following a diet plan, the dieter will be open to eating anything that can't run and hide (actually I have been known to eat some run-and-hide food items too).*

*Theory number two—refer back to theory number one—where's Freud when you need him?*

*Personal experience has taught me that this theory is most certainly evidence based. After a few weeks of expert discipline and control while following a regimented plan, I can eat undeterred and indiscriminately for days, weeks, and sometimes years at a stretch. This, my dear thin friend is where your weight gain will start. Trust me. After your dieting weeks, nothing will keep you from food. My experience has been that during these moments of heightened food awareness following dieting, not even Daniel Day Lewis (loin cloth and all running through the woods as the last Mohican) could distract me from food (although I would invite him to eat with me).*

# The road to hell is paved with sugar

Still focused on weight and thankfully able to have a sense of humor about the futility of my food behavior, a few months passed before I recorded more angst over food. This time I revisited the sugar problem.

<u>March 3, 2000</u>

I've been reading about nutrition and disease and aging. I believe my moods and sleepiness are sugar related. I believe I would be much happier and more energetic if I quit sugar and refined carbohydrates altogether. It's not easy to change but I believe it is in my best interest. I'm hoping to start now.

<u>March 5, 2000</u>

I've had a good 24 hour fast. This is a good time to quit sugar. Wish me luck. Help!

Finally after months of severe fatigue, lethargy, and depression, I sought medical advice and with a simple blood test was diagnosed with a non-functioning thyroid. Finally I had a physiological reason for my fatigue and weight gain. Certainly now with medication correction I would be able to lose weight. I had visions of being size six by summer. I even took more of the thyroid medication than prescribed and when I had repeat blood work my doctor looked alarmed. I sheepishly said that I was not following the dose as prescribed. I had been taking extra hoping to expedite my thinness. You'd think that a nurse ought to know better. Such was the desperation I felt to be thin, but thin did not come.

<u>May 21, 2000</u>

I had a medical physical last week and got weighed—176 pounds. Yikes! I don't know what was worse, standing on the scale or getting a pap smear. I'm taking thyroxin now for a non-functioning thyroid. Perhaps that's part of my weight problem. I'm not sure why this is such an issue with me, but I really would like to be thin. Now I've got all these size eight clothes from Hawaii that I can't wear.

Frustration escalates as I look longingly at the closet full of clothes that I can no longer wear. Summer had arrived and none of my summer 1999 clothes fit. This journal entry reflects again the despair I felt over weight problems.

<u>June 27, 2000</u>

I'm grieving the loss of my slim body. As I look in my closet at the size eight to ten summer clothes I wore last year I want to cry. Why, why, why couldn't I maintain that size with all the exercise I get?

I'm trying to recapture my confidence in being able to get the fat off again. Go away my hopeless attitude. Failure is only failure when you stop trying. It's like there are two people living in my body. One has all control and wants to eat only nutritious food. The other one can't stop eating junk food. The battle of the spirit continues. Will the good defeat the junk? Can I shrink this huge gap between who I am and who I want to be? For Heaven's sake! I'm 44 years old and I'm struggling with the same weight and food obsession I had in my twenties.

What I want is to be lean, muscular, and fit. I believe that I am muscular and fit because of my regular exercise, but there are so many mounds of fat on my muscle that no one but me can tell.

I bought a new bike last week, an 18-speed, and biked out to the wildlife center—must be over ten miles. I consider myself quite fit to be able to bike ten miles in ninety minutes when I haven't biked since leaving Hawaii ten months ago. I know my muscles are in good form. I'm not sore. The day after biking to the wildlife center, I biked to my sister's and back—that's ten miles. I'm an athlete for Heaven's sake! Why am I so fat?

Walking and cycling my way through the summer and fall months failed to reduce my weight. On the contrary, it continued to climb to the end of the year.

November 24, 2000

I'm still fat. I finally gave all my skinny clothes to my sister so I didn't have to be depressed looking at them.

In the local newspaper I read an ad for a spiritually based weight loss program and grabbed on to the hope that this might be my ultimate solution. With girth expanding while eating my way through the rest of the year, I hopefully fantasized about this new program I would join in the New Year. All would be well if I could just get through the year and into a new weight loss program.

December 4, 2000

I bought a grey fleece extra-large skirt and an olive colored big sweater. Help! I'm getting bigger and bigger. I'm joining Weigh Down in January to get some help.

December 26, 2000

I ate fattening goodies at work. Ugh! Poisoned pup syndrome.

December 27, 2000

I ate at Mr. Mike's in Cranbrook and ate too much as usual. I'm bigger than I've ever been and trying to psych myself up for a major behavior change to get rid of all this excess fat. I can't believe how fat I've become. I've grown out of the fat clothes I bought a couple months ago. When will it end? I really do want to be thin. I know I can beat this food habit. I know I can.

December 31, 2000

Here I am again sitting by the fire at the close of another day and year. I just read last year's resolutions. Unfortunately they've not been accomplished.

Not only did I not lose weight this year, I actually gained about thirty pounds. I weighed myself at work this week—204 pounds! Ouch. This is more than I weighed nine months pregnant. I can't believe I've got myself so fat again. But here I face another year still carrying my old habits, optimistic still that I will overcome.

So here I am with more of the same goals to write. This will be the year I beat my weight battle.

I want to weigh 130 pounds by this time next year.

In retrospect, I wonder if my obsession over weight was a means of taking the focus off the marriage and family turmoil I was experiencing. I had teenagers now and worried immensely about them. I felt terribly isolated in this as well as in an unhealthy marriage that I seemed helpless to heal. If that wasn't enough, I was working on courses to complete a university degree.

It's a mystery to me now that I did not stop all this madness and work on the troubled relationships in my life and sit down for a good honest discussion with the people in my intimate circle. That was frightening to me. I ate conflicts away rather than face them and try to resolve them. It was easier to deny and avoid any problems and just eat. Certainly that could make everything all better.

Stuck in all this turmoil that seemed beyond my capacity to handle, I turned to what always seemed to give me the love and comfort I was missing in my life. If I could just be thin, I fantasized that I could then cope well with whatever else was going awry in my quickly unravelling marriage.

One thing for sure was that I needed help beyond my ability to cope, from a Power much greater than myself.

# Pray down and up again

New hopes emerged as I set out for group support focusing on a spiritual approach to weight loss. I had always believed in God, so this seemed to be a natural fit for my natural woman problem.

Many of my journal entries for this year reflect the spiritual approach learned in Weigh Down as I attempted to apply this approach to my weight problem. A major tenet of this program is to eat whatever you want as long as you are physically hungry and eat only the amount needed to stop the hunger. When the eating monster rears its ugly head, a turn to God is the recommended intervention.

Certainly by now I knew that I needed a miracle to conquer my problem. As with other weight loss plans, it worked initially while I was in the honeymoon phase of the plan.

January 15, 2001

I want to eat, but I don't want to eat. That's another symptom of the larger problem, eating to excess. Last night I went to an orientation for the Weigh Down workshop and I hope to embrace the principles to control my body's size.

Another journal entry clearly shows my habit of turning to food whenever I feel stumped in life.

January 18, 2001

I am working on a paper. As soon as I got stumped and didn't know what to write, I started eating and basically kept eating until bedtime. Why? Why? Why?

Today I start again. My life is filled with starting points. Please help me God. I don't want to be trapped in food hell and fat hell for the rest of my life. I'm an intelligent, strong woman. I should be able to conquer this. If nothing else this year, help me defeat my fat hell demons. Whatever it is that food does for me, rather than make me fat, help me find out and overcome it.

During this time I was taking a university nutrition course for my nursing degree and found it quite motivating. I recalled the many fad diets I had followed in the past decades: fit for life, Atkins, zone, south beach, rotation diet, carbohydrate addict's diet, grapefruit diets, fat free diets, sugar free diets, liquid diets, solid food diets, seven day diets, two day diets, two hour diets, and on and on and on, ad nauseam. The nutrition course, in a sense, brought me back to my diet senses and to the moderation of eating whole food, or so it seemed for a while.

January 25, 2001

After studying my nutrition course I'm back to eating low fat, hi fiber with an abundance of fruit and veggies – the Word of Wisdom (*Doctrine and Covenants* section 89). I should have stuck with that all along instead of following the fads. God is always right. I'm praying daily for help with my appetite and weight. I want to weigh 130 pounds by the end of 2001.

My sincere desire for spirituality and goodness is reflected numerous times in my journals. I spent my time reading motivating literature and wanting to be a better person. My spirit really was willing but my fat flesh seemed weak and rebellious.

February 13, 2001

I must conquer my flesh if I am to progress to greater spiritual heights. Overcoming physical temptation is a must in order to progress. I am whole-heartedly working on this with regards to excess food. Greed is a sin that I have been guilty of through overeating. Food is not love; God is love. I am turning to God to help me overcome. After years of leaning on man's advice through diet books and various gadgets I am turning to God with full purpose.

I pray several times daily to overcome this temptation and I believe I will overcome. I will leave the worship of food behind me and pursue God with all my heart.

February 15, 2001

It snowed heavily this morning. I walked in the snow. I'm feeling positive and optimistic about overcoming my weakness to overeat. I'm having good success with prayer and focusing on God rather than food. I will weigh 130 pounds before this year is over.

It is unfortunate that I cannot locate the Weigh Down workbooks I filled while laboring over weight during this year. I may have destroyed them or someone else may have destroyed them or they were simply and mistakenly cast off. To think that I could have had pages and pages and pages more of my neurotic relationship with food to immortalize in this book! As it is I only have the journal entries alluding to such a workbook during this time.

<u>February 23, 2001</u>

I've been doing the Weigh Down thing and writing in the workbook my thoughts on overcoming sin. I'm doing well.

<u>March 4, 2001</u>

I had a good walk this morning before church. I'm sitting by the fire enjoying the warmth. I'm happy to fit back into my fat suits, so I've downsized from high risk obese to obese. Next will be chubby, then average, and then lean. Yippee, Skippy, it's working again. I'm losing weight. I feel liberated with the thought of eating whatever I want as long as I'm genuinely hungry and not eating 'til I'm full.

<u>March 13, 2001</u>

I feel that the burden of overeating is gone from me. God has replaced the love of food with love for Him.

<u>May 30, 2001</u>

I'm doing another twelve-week session of the Weigh Down workshop. I'm convinced that feasting on the words of Christ is much better than feasting on food to fill me up spiritually. Since the end of January when I first started I have not had a pig out. That is amazing to me.

The highs of the initial Weigh Down program seemed to plunge sometime in the summer of 2001 as family difficulties continued to plague me. I felt terribly alone in my struggles with marriage and family. It seemed to challenge me daily as I tried to regroup and refocus.

September 6, 2001

I've gotta refocus and write again the goals I had for this year. Get down to 130 pounds.

September 25, 2001

I went to a Weigh Down meeting last night, the first one for the fall. I'm glad I went. It was nice to refocus on goals. I found it motivating.

The fall of 2001 was unbearably turbulent for me. My son in grade seven was suspended from school and I opted to homeschool him for the remainder of the year. I felt that he had been unjustly treated by the school administration and for a time I nurtured the disdain I held for the principal as I watched the misery and loneliness it caused for my son who had been so eager to be off to another school year.

As I worked on my own university courses I helped him with his school, feeling sadness daily for him and the sports opportunities he was missing by being home-schooled.

Add to that turmoil continuing marriage problems and angst over teen children and I had a recipe for binging. Eating to hide myself from my misery continued as a means to cope with the problems I seemed totally inept at addressing and resolving. My fall journal is filled with angst over my family rather than my weight. I ate and cried and worried and prayed and ate and cried and worried and ate and cried and worried. The more I worried, the more I ate and the worse I felt. It was the fall from hell.

# Hell hath no fury like a woman on a diet

By the time 2002 rolled around I was back to recording my efforts at weight management. One brief entry reminds me that I was still trying to solve my food issues with the Weigh Down program.

February 11, 2002

I'm sitting in the Church of God parking lot as I wait for the Weigh Down meeting to start.

The next entry confirms that the monster is still there as I desperately try to understand it.

March 6, 2002

Heavy snowfall yesterday and today. I ate terribly both days and can't seem to fill up and stop. Why is this part of me back? Every time I feel like I've beat it, it comes back to haunt me. It's like there are too many people living in my body fighting for character traits or some such thing. I'm stuffed and disgusted and still wanting to shovel in food. Luckily I'm up at the church while the kids play basketball and there's no food here. I'd really like to go to a dry-out center for bingers or some such thing and fast for days with massage and other treatments to pamper me.

No magical spa or dry-out center appeared to rescue me. I continued to be me, now with three teenagers in the house and a rapidly deteriorating marriage. The next entry only hints at my feelings of yet again another failure.

<u>April 5, 2002</u>

The months go by so fast and I'm always thinking about the weight I could have lost had I remained spiritually oriented and followed my body's true hunger signals. Ah well. Size six, the impossible dream.

So much angst occurred in the spring and summer of 2002 as I made plans to move somewhere, hoping that it would be beneficial to my children's development. They were my life priority and I worried immensely over their development in a town that seemed to idolize booze.

I secured a job in California and packed up my children once again to relocate, forgetting how traumatic and stressful it had been the previous move to Hawaii. I am still not sure why I made this move, which lasted only a few days before I was back home again.

I was clearly floundering and not sure how to deal with the escalating marital problems in my life. About this time my then husband made it known that he wanted separation and divorce. Just what that would look like had not been discussed. Both of us reverted to silent avoidance, perhaps waiting for the other to make the first move. I wanted to salvage and heal what could be healed in the relationship through therapy and reconciliation, he didn't. No constructive discussions occurred, just stony silence, weeks of stony silence as I ate the angst away.

October 4, 2002

Stony silence and tension continue on the home front. I deal with it by eating—my more negative coping mechanism. I just eat myself into a coma so I don't feel anything. I really do need to make a constructive move to deal with the situation, but the fact is I'm scared of him. I feel very intimidated and put down by him.

Avoidance and denial that my marriage was done seemed to work for a while. I kept going day by day, obsessing about my weight in the face of what really was a much greater challenge. Perhaps the weight obsession saved me from facing what really needed to be faced. A coward in my heart and unable to cope, I simply avoided and ignored the situation. It seemed for a time that he did as well.

October 5, 2002

I bought some clothes yesterday. I am so fat again. Hanging in at around size sixteen—literally a round size sixteen. Why, why, why? Why can I not beat this demon of excessive eating? I feel like a butterball all over again—triple chin, triple butt, triple belly and thighs. Why, why, why? I've had about thirty years of this obsession. Up, down, up, down, up down, up down, up up up! Ah well.

I really want to be slim. I went for a walk with some friends last week. It's our unofficial first wives club. My friend separated from her husband a year ago and has dropped what appears to be a ton of weight. She was sort of like me over the past few years, dieting up and down. Now she's so thin. She says that after leaving her husband the stress in her life went down 100% so she no longer ate to reduce stress. Maybe that could happen to me. I couldn't believe how skinny she is. Even her ample butt is gone completely and she weighs around 115 pounds, Holy cow! Could that happen to me? I so want to beat this fat problem.

Here I am working on a master's degree in wellness promotion and I'm eating myself into a coma to cope with the stress. That is so unhealthy.

October 20, 2002

Yesterday I had two four-mile walks, morning and evening. I felt great except that I've really packed on a lot of fat these past few months. I'm not packing on anymore. I am making a change. I will change my mind to change my life. I am going to beat this depressing cycle of weight gain and weight loss and weight gain. I'm going to get lean and fit and look and feel great. I am in control of my mind, my body, and my spirit.

I feel good. I started doing weights again. I'm planning on two walks a day for awhile to get some weight off fast. I'm not healthy at this weight. I know that.

October 23, 2002

It's a beautiful fall day. I went for a lovely walk with a friend. She loaned me a book on fitness, *Body for Life*, to help keep me motivated to get lean. I'm exercising lots and eating moderately. I'm going to beat this fat. I am doing what I need to do to get the fat off and build muscle and bone.

No matter what book or what plan or what diet from whatever or whomever, it just couldn't fix the misery in my soul or my life.

# The sounds of binging

Silence didn't really solve anything. It's very hard to share a life with someone who hates you. I felt as low as I had ever felt before and continued only to go through the motions of family life for the love of my precious children.

November 6, 2002

More tension. More conflict.

The monster is back, the one I've been fighting for thirty years—the eating monster. So many times I've thought I had it beat, but no, it's back again. I feel insecure, scared, disorganized, ugly, and sad all at the same time. What hole is food going to fill?

The depth and breadth of the dark hole of divorce was something I had not anticipated. How can you know the depths of hell if you have never been there? In my journal I tried to understand myself in the context of failing at marriage. My anger and frustration at hiding myself with food rather than living my authentic life is very much evident as I rant in this middle of the night entry.

November 10, 2002 1:40 a.m.

I feel like my world is falling apart or perhaps it never was together. That was just a lie I concocted to protect myself. Now the truth comes out. It always does. I feel like I've been pretending all my life, playing roles that I think I am expected to play. Now I want to play me but the question is, who am I if it isn't all those other roles I've been filling?

I feel like what I want has never been acknowledged or honored by myself or by anyone else. But how can I expect anyone else to honor me when I don't honor myself? To thine own self be true. What am I afraid of? Why can't I say what I really feel? For years I've been denying who I really am. What am I afraid of? I really have nothing to hide, so why have I always been afraid to be who I really am? There's no need to pretend to be someone else. No more pretence, no more denial. No more stuffing the truth with food. The truth will not be stuffed. It will not go away (neither will the fat that I've accumulated by trying to make it go away). Coming to grips with who I am—is that Ruth Blackmore, Ruth Boehmer, Ruth Perrin, Ruth something else? The Moabite? The "whither thou goest" woman? I will go where I will go, no more following someone else's path. I will blaze my own trail with the *Book of Mormon* as my guide.

I'm packing about sixty extra pounds of someone else's life on my body. I'm not packing anyone else anymore. Get off my back, my butt, my belly, my chin, my chest, my thighs—get off me.

From where the sun now sets, I will fake no more forever. I will have a voice. I will honor my voice. I will be true to myself first.

In mid-November 2002 my then husband moved out and the legal hell of divorce began.

Thankfully my love of walking was right up there with my love of eating and provided me with the peace I craved on a daily basis. When fear gripped me I went out for a walk.

<u>November 24, 2002</u>

I am thankful that my body is strong enough to take me out on a five mile walk every day. I'm thankful for my walking habit and the great peace it brings to me. There are few things that uplift my spirits like a brisk outdoor walk. Some days if I wake up feeling blue I just tie on my shoes and head outside. Just the simple act of stepping outside lifts my spirits. I'm convinced that the Spirit is in the trees, the air, the mountains, and sky and when I'm outside, it is in me too. That's how I feel.

<u>December 30, 2002</u>

I really want to get rid of my food excesses. I really want to conquer that this year. I was talking to a colleague at work on Boxing Day. She has lost eighty pounds since January 2002 doing low fat and daily exercise.

Another year ended and I was still fat. Besides being fat, now I was going through a divorce. There I was, still obsessing and dreaming about that elusive size that would give me the perfect life whatever that was.

# My coat of many sizes

Another year came and with it new hopes for a good year, *good* being defined as getting thin. The first journal entry for the year shows again my desire and goal to be thin. I love that I have a sense of humor about many of my personal human struggles and can still have a laugh during emotionally turbulent times. I was always such a great starter, but alas, not a great finisher – at least not with weight challenges.

January 1, 2003

I'm visualizing what I would like a year from now. I see myself lean, like 130 pounds lean and fit. I was going to give up swearing but right now it's my crutch while I give up sugar and excess food.

One day down, 364 to go.

I seemed to have all the knowledge for change but somehow never quite changed. My positive affirmations in the next journal entry attest to my belief in positive self-talk. I had read many times that if you can see it you can be it; if you can think it you can be it. Had I not thought and visualized and thought and visualized and thought and visualized myself damn near into a coma? What could I be missing still? The truth is that somewhere between seeing and being is a whole helluva lot of sweating and probably swearing too.

January 2, 2003

Heavy snow. I walked six miles in heavy snow then did a weight workout.

I love my body. I treat it with honor and reverence as a temple. I eat only what is good for my body. I care for myself. I am balanced and at peace with myself.

10:00 p.m. I walked another six miles this evening.

Looking back now, it seems rather overly optimistic that I would solve my eating problems in the year I was going through the hell of divorce, yet there it is in writing, my fantasy that this would be the year for me. I should at least get a medal for my tenacity and hope in the face of seemingly insurmountable thighs. Oh, screw medals! All I wanted was to be thin.

January 4, 2003

I walked six miles yesterday and today. I am confident that this is my year to conquer my poor eating habits, to balance my life and really shine.

January 5, 2003 Wt. 188 pounds.

I walked four miles.

I'm going to weigh myself once a month on Sunday.

Evening: I walked another four miles.

February 2, 2003

I was so disappointed to stand on the scale and have lost only four pounds in a month. I wanted to cry but didn't have time because I had to get to work.

May 16, 2003

I am doing well with exercising and eating. I am down twenty pounds since Christmas. I am feeling good and feeling positive.

In June, 2003 my oldest child graduated from high school and began searching for what she would do with her adult life. I stressed and worried about her, knowing that having parents separate and divorce during her final year of high school made for a very stressful and sad year for her. This was yet another trigger for me to eat the guilt I was feeling for failing at marriage and family.

In the summer of 2003 I finally moved out of the family home, taking my children with me. I got a teaching job in Spokane, Washington and moved my children there. Those months were filled with terrible grief and loneliness and for the second time in my life I genuinely lost my appetite and could not eat. I had heard people (usually my skinny friends and sisters) talk of having no appetite and not being able to eat, but this was a phenomenon that I simply had not understood. What do you mean you can't eat? Just pick up the damn food, put it in your mouth, chew and swallow, I would think. Now it had hit me and in my incapacitating grief, I could not eat.

By the time fall came, I was relatively slim, slimmer than I had been in a number of years. In my grief and the grief of my children, the move to Spokane was aborted and we returned again to the familiar comfort of Creston. Back in Creston it dawned on me that I was slim. I hadn't really noticed this until then. My journal indicates the positive feelings I had about my size as well as the commitment to keep the weight off.

October 14, 2003

I'm quite comfortable in my size right now—size ten jeans. It feels good to have the excess weight gone again. I'm going to stay very focused on keeping it off this time.

November 25, 2003

I weigh 145 pounds. I've lost almost fifty pounds so far this year and it feels absolutely wonderful. I can't believe how fun it is to no longer be fat. I've bought a wonderful wardrobe of Ralph Lauren jackets, lovely sweaters, and jeans. Some size ten, some size eight. It feels so great. I hope I never get fat again. I look good. I feel good. I feel optimistic about my future here.

Thankfully in December 2003 I secured a job teaching practical nursing students for a year. At last I would not have the torture of shift work for a time. Things seemed to be working out for me after the year from hell. I purchased a home for my family and prepared to move in in the New Year. Being slim was just the icing off the cake.

## Oh scale, where is thy victory?

Finally I had a year to celebrate some goals achieved. It seemed that I had arrived and felt comfortable with my achievement.

January 1, 2004

Looking over my goals from last January, I see that I have accomplished a few: I'm forty pounds less this year than last.

March 28, 2004

I'm thinking how nice it is to not be fat anymore. I feel lovely and slim. It's a great feeling—far better than any food binge could be. I love being leaner and I hope to get even leaner and fitter this year.

It did not take long into the year before I realized that my food demons had once again resurfaced. Relieved as I was not to feel the crippling fear and grief I had the previous year, I did not appreciate the return of my appetite.

April 15, 2004

I had a good Easter. I had a dinner here. I ate way too much and am still on a bad sugar trip.

With the return of my appetite came the return of weight obsessing and searching for the ultimate solution.

April 21, 2004

I just got back from a church women's meeting. It was incredible. The guest speaker spoke on obesity and healthy weight management. She's lost 120 pounds in the past couple years and related much of her own personal journey. It was incredibly motivating and boosted my spirits a hundred fold.

May 1, 2004

I feel very healthy this morning. I had a long bike ride last night then ate some fresh strawberries for a snack.

May 29, 2004

I had a good day of eating fruit only. I needed to do something to get me off the binge train again. I seriously don't want to get fat again. I really want to keep control of my weight. I feel I'm back in control after today and I'm going to get down more weight. I bought a new skirt today, size eleven. Some of my pants are getting snug again so I want to get back to loose pants.

I'd like to get down to size six, being ultra-fit.

During 2004 I walked regularly a gruelling uphill climb near my home, and yet by the end of the year my weight had climbed over twenty pounds and my clothes no longer fit. How could that be? I must admit to some rather bitter feelings every time I stood in the grocery store line-up and looked at all those glossy magazines headlining walking programs for walking off ten, twenty, thirty, forty pounds. In the bitterness of my fat I would think, I walk more than anyone else I know and I am fat! By all accounts, according to what the *experts* on walking were saying, I should weigh about twenty pounds by now. But **I'm** not bitter!

Whether thin or fat, I clearly recognized the mood elevating qualities of regular walking.

> December 25, 2004
>
> I'm not sure how I keep up with the pace of my life and not get sick. I believe that my habits of daily walking, scripture reading, and prayer have greatly contributed to this. I'm thankful that my health is holding out through my trouble. I recently had a complete physical/blood work/cholesterol and all that stuff. My doctor tells me that I have the cardiac profile of an athlete. All that hiking up the steep hills here is paying off.

Much as my blood profile was fit, I still lamented the outward appearance of not being fit. I was again, by all accounts, about thirty pounds over what may be deemed healthy for my height. It's enough to drive a food junkie to eat. And that's what I did.

At this point my teaching contract came to a close and I was once again dependent on shift work at the hospital. Ouch! Double ouch! I smell a binge coming on.

# Dieting is not for the faint of heart

The year 2005 brought a first for me. It was the first time I had joined Weight Watchers. After years of hearing colleagues and friends discuss their meetings, I finally decided to join. Strangely I had known only one or two people who had had any long time success with Weight Watchers, but that was good enough for me. It was better than the success I had had with any of my previous dieting plans.

January 2, 2005

Now the holiday season is done and I've got to get the oomph to get going with some new goals. Actually they're the same old goals. My old food demons came back so I've got to shake them again.

February 27, 2005

I joined Weight Watchers two weeks ago. I lost five pounds the first week. I'll have my second weigh in on Tuesday. I hope last night's pig-out hasn't tainted my results.

I had two major hill hikes today so maybe I'll work it off between now and then. Maybe two hours of exercise tomorrow and Tuesday will save me.

March 22, 2005

I continue to go to Weight Watchers. I have lost eleven pounds in the first four weeks. Tonight is my weigh in for the fifth week.

Spring 2005

I would feel liberated if I knew that excess of eating would never be part of my life again, if I knew that I would never eat except in response to hunger and always stop when hunger was met.

April 5, 2005

I only lost a fifth of a pound at weigh in. I'm down 12.7 pounds in seven weeks. I signed up for the next ten weeks and hope to lose another fifteen pounds.

I had three long uphill walks today.

I had continuing stress with single parenting teens, working full time, and trying to pay all the bills associated with children, school, sports, mortgage, and so forth. Then my eighteen year old son had an emergency appendectomy, sending me over the edge with food again.

May 2, 2005

For some reason I had a major eating attack yesterday and couldn't seem to control it. I haven't had one that bad in a long time.

May 4, 2005

I feel happy and grateful for my life. I got my spiritual self filled up again so the eating frenzy stopped.

May 9, 2005

I have a closet full of lovely clothes, more than I've ever owned in my life. Being slim makes clothes more fun.

May 22, 2005

I bought some Capri pants for work and more tops and three pairs of shoes. I admit it seems a bit excessive, but I'm enjoying so much being a more attractive size ten rather than the sixteen and eighteen I used to be.

I went to Weight Watchers. I am happy to have lost a total of twenty pounds since starting in February.

Happy indeed, but once again it did not last. As usual every diet worked as long as I worked it, but exactly how long could I work them? It seemed not very long and certainly not permanently. How could I continue to justify spending so much money just to lose weight that would inevitably come back again?

All that dieting and weight-watching just reaffirmed that I was a failure. With my ever-changing sizes, all the community could see it too. There's no place to hide when you're constantly changing sizes and shapes and on display for your little world to see. It gives a whole new meaning to being a fat frog in a little pond.

Alas, it goes without saying that I never did get a life-time membership in Weight Watchers, nor did I become their poster girl or spokesperson or success story.

May 24, 2005

I feel like I'm flying apart again and wanting to eat out of control. I'm feeling afraid and overwhelmed by life. I seem to have this wave hit me once in awhile. I don't know if it's related to hormones or what but I'm struggling again with fear of handling finances and raising children.

Yesterday I worked twelve hours at the hospital. As the day went and I got more and more tired I kind of fell apart and ate candies, cake etc. I felt exhausted, blue, scared, and everything else.

Once again I was suffering from post-diet stress disorder. The binging continued as I frantically looked for an alternative solution to my perennial problem.

# Thigh to thigh

Sometime in the spring of 2005 I was introduced to a twelve-step program for food addicts. This program was based on a scriptural foundation for the twelve steps patterned after alcoholics anonymous. A small group of women in my church community had started the program in Creston. I happened to have overheard them discussing it at church and my ears perked up at the sound of weight loss. My ever-optimistic spirit was certain that this was the new solution I so needed. I was excited to once again focus on a spiritual approach to my chronic weight problem.

June 14, 2005

Food thoughts in our little food group. This week
we discussed our food woes and compulsion to eat.
I pondered this as I thought of times that I've given
in to unhealthy food amounts. Food in its original
purpose is to nurture and strengthen but when used to
excess it becomes a weapon for destruction.

I suppose I could add that food in its natural form and purpose really can be a weapon for mass destruction. I eternally hoped that it would destroy a few pounds of my mass, but instead the mass would leave for a while then always return somehow, not really destroyed at all. I have heard it said that matter can neither be created nor destroyed, so the mass I carry has to go somewhere and stay off of me when I lose it; otherwise it is always out there somewhere floating around waiting to come back. I don't really care where it goes. I just wish it would stay there. Wherever the mass was, it was gone for another milestone in my life.

My second child graduated in 2005 and I was relieved to be relatively slim for the graduation grand march with him. I had survived getting a second teen through high school and the cesspool of Creston teen life. With the continuing changes in my family life, I clung to whatever felt secure for me—usually food. So the summer of 2005 passed with me binging, praying, fasting, binging, praying, fasting, binging, praying, and fasting some more.

I continued on in my twelve-step work.

June 29, 2005

I went to the food addiction meeting and came away more resolved to seek God continually to help conquer my sins. I'm going to more fully make an attempt to use the tools daily. Writing is one of them.

I'm going to use food only for hunger and not for love or hate or solace or stress or anything else.

Who was I trying to kid? Not using food for love or hate or solace or stress? How could I survive without my crutch? What would I do when life continued on reminding me of my biggest failure in life, my marriage? How could I cope if I could not numb the pain and guilt and fear with food?

July 3, 2005

After attending a bridal shower for my nephew's fiancé I had a bad eating spell both at the shower and later at home. I feel like an abnormal nobody that doesn't fit in any society.

July 6, 2005

I went on three walks today so I've had over three hours of vigorous exercise. I should be rail thin. I went to the food addiction meeting. It's always good to share honestly my feelings, fears, concerns.

July 10, 2005

I am deeply grateful for my physical health—that I can run and walk and cycle—and all my muscles, bones, and body parts communicate with each other and operate smoothly. I am deeply grateful for the joy of physical activity and the powerful mood elevator that it is.

July 13, 2005

I've already been out for a two hour bike ride through Canyon and Lister, about fifteen miles. I biked all the way up my hill—what an athlete. I wonder why I weigh as much as I do. Of course it would have something to do with the ice-cream I had last night.

August 3, 2005

I feel terribly hung-over from sugar. I made chocolate chip cookies last night, thinking my boys needed some home baked treats. Of course I ate more cookies than anyone. Now I feel sick and headachy. Will I ever learn?

August 13, 2005

I had a lovely walk then a 2 ½ hour bike ride this morning. Now it's 6:40 p.m. and I'm just getting ready to go to work for four hours. I felt a little bummed this evening and ate some cookies. Not sure what the feeling was, maybe tired, maybe rebellious, maybe frightened, maybe not. I really don't know. I just felt a bit low.

August 28, 2005

I'm deeply blessed right now to not be fat. I feel the strength of God lifting me above the burden and bondage of food addiction.

I'm blessed with a tremendously strong healthy body and a desire to move—walk, run, hike, cycle.

Besides my own children, I frequently had others living and staying and camping and eating, and whatever else kids do when they don't have a home or don't want to go to their home. Anyway, I frequently had a child's friend or cousin or two staying over. This sometimes added to my stress and eating level.

August 31, 2005

I was all hyped to go biking and set out on my bike. I didn't have to change gears until I got to the uphill by the reserve (about five miles), then the gears thing broke and I was stranded and had to walk back pushing the bike. I was so upset because my sons' friends have been riding my bike and doing stupid things like jumping. I fumed most of the way home planning to have a screaming fit and throw everyone out. I didn't. I baked bread and cookies instead.

I went to the food addiction meeting tonight. We're reading the overeater's anonymous book together. It's a wonderful book, so plain and honest.

When my oldest son moved away to work I felt an emptiness and sadness that sent me back into food hell, attempting to fill the hole that his moving left in my mother's heart.

September 15, 2005

I don't know what's wrong with me. I'm stuffed from binge eating candy and popcorn. What's wrong with me? I know sugar is terrible for me. I really crashed today.

I am still not sure what the answer to that desperate question is. I continued to plan and diet and set goals and ruminate and cogitate and masticate and meditate and medicate with food and on and on and on.

# The more thighs change, the more they stay the same

After launching my second child out into the world, it was back to life raising two more teens. I spent many weekends watching their sports games, which brought the awkward moments of being around their father.

Being around my former husband always brought out the old self-loathing insecurities that I felt living with him. I felt like a low life failure when in his presence. With the feelings of worthlessness came the feeding frenzies I loathed so much.

<u>September 17, 2005</u>

Last night I had a feeding frenzy worse than any for months. I don't know what got into me. Today I am feeling tense having to be in the same room as my ex-husband watching volleyball games.

As the days of binging continued, I set out a plan of writing down all food intake, moods, times, and amounts to hopefully remedy the situation before the weight came back. I think I already knew what triggered eating frenzies; I just couldn't seem to divert them. After a few weeks of food recording I tossed that tool to the wind too.

<u>September 30, 2005</u>

I'm eating myself into oblivion again. It seems like the .....

That last entry ended abruptly. I must have been distracted (food?) and never got back to finish that thought. Let me guess, it probably said the more I try not to eat, the more I eat? If it wasn't so pathetic and hadn't caused me so much personal misery and torment, I could laugh myself slim just looking at the rapidly swinging food pendulum in my life, from all to nothing and back again faster than you can eat a bag of chips. It makes me dizzy just reading about the swinging moods and foods.

<u>October 6, 2005</u>

I am absolutely stuffed—ugh! The monster is back. I have not yet humbled myself. I know I am harboring sadness and regret over past mistakes. I was so insensitive. I know I want to apologize in person and I have to do it in order to let go of some of my pain.

Some personal things in this journal should not be published so I have left some blanks to protect the privacy of certain people in my life. That and I really don't want to disclose all my pathetic neuroticism. Some things have to be left unsaid, just as some food has to be left uneaten if that is at all possible.

# Fat frustrated and fifty

Closing in on fifty I sat down to do another life inventory. My life inventories actually meant weight inventories. There I was at fifty, still battling my food demons. That which I feared most had come upon me—fat! On my fiftieth birthday I penned these goals, my forty day plan for change:

October 9, 2005

Have a plan—(October 10-November 18)

This is my forty day plan to jolt myself back to God where food addiction is concerned.

1. Eat only in response to hunger
2. Eat only in amounts to take hunger away
3. Phone more, three times a week to connect with twelve-step members

This is my plan of action for when temptation strikes with its cunning powerful and baffling force:

1. pray sincerely
2. use the tools, remember them, commit them to memory
3. go to the piano and play
4. write out my feelings, cry if necessary

> The closer I get to God, the farther I am from temptation.

I'm not sure why I had set a forty day plan as if there was some magic in forty days. I probably read another one of those useless self-help books that claimed if you could do something for forty days you were set in a new habit. Well it looks more like it's gonna take forty years. Wait a minute, it already HAS! I don't need another self-help book, I need God's help.

Sure enough, the forty day plan aborted prematurely. Only two weeks later the monster had returned and the goals were abandoned to the pull of food hell. At this time I had a sixteen year old son and a thirteen year old daughter living at home. My life revolved around their sports, church, and school activities, while my mind revolved around my weight issues.

You gotta hand it to me; I was tenacious in my attempts and still hopeful that the dream was out there somewhere.

<u>October 25, 2005</u>

> Why am I descending into food hell again? I'm feeling overwhelmed and scared again. I don't know why. Every time I think those feelings are gone they come back again. Sometimes I wish I could just have a really good cry when it comes on and maybe I could feel better.
>
> I feel like I'm empty or scattered or confused or something on the edge. I'm really not sure, but the old crutch food comes back to torment me. I want this bondage to be gone.

A day later I took pen in hand to carve out my goals for abstinence from compulsive overeating. At this point I felt that making amends (step nine) was something I needed to do in order to conquer the eating monster. It seemed that my torment over past mistakes was eating me up in the same megabites I was eating up food. The mistakes I had made in marriage haunted me day and night, leaving me filled with self-loathing and stuffing myself with food to hide from the pain of remorse and regret.

I couldn't change the past. I knew that. I also knew that I had to take responsibility for my mistakes and let it go. I knew that only God could give me the strength to make amends face to face with the person I had most harmed. My journal entries are a blend of planning, praying, pleading, and placing my name in favorite scripture verses.

October 26, 2005

Once again I'm committing myself to the tools of the twelve-step recovery program. Following our weekly meeting tonight, I'm feeling positive in making this renewed commitment.

The plan: abstain from sugar and all junk food:

- eat balanced meals fruit/protein/ complex carbohydrates/nuts/seeds
- drink a minimum of ten cups of water daily
- think the plan, work through the daily reading of the program, and memorize the daily scripture. Keep it in my thoughts.

When temptation hits:

a. pray
b. read

c. write
d. phone
e. feel what I need to feel
f. Make amends to a person before next Wednesday and report at the meeting.

Father in Heaven: Thank you for my dear supportive friends. Thank you for this magnificent body. Please help me to treat it with the honor and respect it deserves as the temple of my eternal soul. See these goals I have set for this week. I will put forth this effort that I may call upon thy power to help me overcome this destructive food demon in my life. I know that I am powerless over my addictions and only with thy power will I overcome. Please give me the power I need, Lord.

October 27, 2005 4:30 a.m.

2 Nephi 9:39 (*Book of Mormon*) Oh Ruth, remember the awfulness in transgressing against that Holy God and the awfulness of yielding to the enticing of that cunning one. Remember to be carnally minded is death and to be spiritually minded is life eternal.

For me, remember how dreadful you feel when you yield to your physical appetite to excess, how awful it feels to over indulge, the anxiety, fear, depression, and resentment that results. Remember the awfulness of gaining weight and not fitting all those lovely clothes in your closet, the awfulness of flatus and having to run away from people because of the smell and embarrassment. I don't want this lifestyle. I want the spiritual lifestyle that brings joy, peace, hope, health, and youth, and enjoying the simplicity of choosing clothes for each day and knowing they fit comfortably and l look good in them.

I want to receive the spiritual gift of a complete loss of desire to eat outside the bounds the Lord has set. I would like the confidence I have in knowing I will never be tempted again to overeat, just like the confidence I have that I will never drink or smoke or do drugs. That's the confidence I'd like to have in regard to food.

October 29, 2005

Just for today. I had an epiphany about this AA quote. I've always been annoyed by it because I would think it really isn't just for today. You can't fool me into believing it's just for today. Finally I was enlightened to realize that it is just for today because each day I resist, I am a stronger person so it's really a different me each day. If I get through this day without my addiction I will be seeing it in a different person the next day.

October 30, 2005

I had a turkey dinner for mom to celebrate her birthday. I didn't pig out. I had one small piece of carrot cake with a tablespoon of ice-cream then stopped.

October 31, 2005

I had a good day at work. Thankfully I felt a bit nauseated and headachy so haven't eaten any excess so far. Thank you God for taking the desire away.

I had chicken and salad for supper with an orange and apple. I am not going to eat, even if it is Halloween and candy is abundant.

<u>November 1, 2005</u>

Praise God for taking me above the Halloween treats that do beset me on all sides at home and at work. Thank you God for keeping me from indulging in them.

# Ghosts of binges past

The pull of the Halloween candy proved to be too strong for my tenuous abstinence as seen in this next entry. Sadly one binge leads to another and another and another until I was actively using my drug of choice once again.

> November 3, 2005
>
> I'm not sure why but I finally caved into Alicia's Halloween candy tonight.
>
> It all started with thinking about the Halloween treats, then I started wanting them, and soon I was eating them.
>
> November 5, 2005
>
> Please redeem me from food addiction hell. I had a binge today while waiting for Gordon's volleyball game. I was stuck in Kimberly feeling bored, restless, a bit tense (my ex-husband was there too), so I ate. I hate myself when I get into that food hell rut.

When conquering food seemed too much to bear, I again added compulsive exercise in the hopes that I could out exercise my bad eating habits. If I could just exercise enough, I fantasized that I could eat whatever I wanted or didn't want but still compulsively ate. I saw the monster as something evil that continued to destroy my peace.

November 7, 2005

I had three walks today and I'm on the worst food binge.

Dear God,

What have I done wrong that this evil is back in my life that I am once again submitting to food hell rather than to thee? Help me, God. I desperately need thy help every minute of every hour of every day. I'm sick and I'm bloated. I've had supper then chocolate chips then a blizzard then a bag of popcorn. I'm desperate. I don't want to be like this. I want that peaceful calm spirit back with no obsession for food. Help me please help me. Lord, please help me stop this destructive habit. What do I need to do that this terrible evil will leave me again?

November 8, 2005 6:45 a.m.

Now here I am again with a food hangover, the awfulness of transgressing food laws. It sure would be a lot easier if I could just live without food all together instead of having to balance it in moderation. I don't want this food hell again. What's wrong with me, Lord? I know that I am powerless over food. Why am I so stubborn and self-destructive? Why? Why do I continue to self-inflict this body and spirit with such impure excess? I know that only thy power can help me.

2 Nephi 4:19 (*Book of Mormon*). "And when I desire to rejoice, my heart groaneth because of my sins." Not only my heart, but my head and stomach and bowels as well. This food excess really wreaks havoc with every system, both carnal and spiritual.

Epiphany: Why is it that I need worldly evidence to support what God has told me (i.e. the sugar thing). I'm lying here reading scripture thinking about how awful I feel and how maybe I should read some worldly research on the connection between sugar and migraines to convince me that it really is not good for me to eat sugar.

Duh! Do I need another study to tell me what my body has been screaming at me for decades?

# Fatter, more frustrated and still fifty

Abstinence from my addiction continued to elude me and I started to analyze in my journals when my worst binges occurred. In short I was attempting to post-mortem my binges. Sleep deprivation definitely contributed to my eating misery and in turn my binging led to more sleep deprivation—a vicious cycle, a veritable treadmill to hell.

> November 9, 2005
>
> I've noticed a pattern: When I haven't got the sleep I need I weaken very badly and start eating late afternoon. I had to be up to go to CPR recertification from 7-10 p.m. There were cookies and I did eat. I was so tired but had to stay awake. Ick!

Thankfully my sense of humor still allowed me to have a laugh at myself and my misery.

> November 10, 2005 7:30 a.m.
>
> Oh! My body groaneth because of my excess of last night. My head poundeth, my belly churneth, my eyes blurreth, and my mind cloudeth. I remember the awfulness of yielding to the enticing of that cunning carnal one—the real cookie monster.

I've had a terrible night, waking frequently, too hot, too thirsty, too bladder-fulleth—Ugh. Why do I do this to my beautiful body and suffer my soul so much? I really am nothing. I really am weak. I desperately need the power of God to overcome my carnal nature. Please change my heart God. I've spent the night groaning, wallowing, and worrying about Gordon's grades, Alicia's teeth, past parenting mistakes. Did I do too much for my children? Did I not do enough? Was I a bad example? Did I smother? Did I neglect? Was I there too much? Was I not there enough? Oooh, my heart groaneth, my spirit laggeth, my conscience seareth, and my thighs increaseth. I'm sure my midlife hormones rageth or derageth or derail or reverseth or I really haven't a clue.

Give me some Excedrin quicketh to stop the head pounding. At least one symptom may disappeareth.

Lord, I desperately need thy power to get dressed and out the door for this day.

6:30 p.m.

God did get me dressed and out the door for my busy day and I've just come in now. I've got the biggest most debilitating migraine I've had in months. Oh Ruth, remember the awfulness in yielding to the enticing of that cunning one. Please God, help me beat this sugar addiction that I may never again be afflicted with it. Stop my stinky thinking that persuades me to again indulge.

Day one: No sugar. Of course that was easy today because of headache and nausea.

<u>November 11, 2005 7:00 a.m.</u>

My remembrance day; to remember the awfulness of eating sugar and excess.

Day two:

10:00 p.m. I watched four volleyball games. I managed with God's help to keep above the urge to eat sugar.

This next entry is so typical of my deceit when it comes to food, saving food supposedly for a family member to have later when I fully intended to eat it all myself. It is also typical of a pattern I have had for years when having guests for dinner. I couldn't wait for the guests to leave so that I could pig out on the leftover dessert. I usually wouldn't eat excess dessert in front of guests, but when they left I ate everything I could get into.

<u>November 13, 2005</u>

I didn't walk; too tired to get up. I had a good fast, ended with a turkey dinner I cooked and shared with friends. I did well until dessert. My friend brought a chocolate pudding layered dessert and I did eat. Bummer. Okay start again Ruth.

Of course I couldn't have just one piece. I indulged secretly by setting aside two pieces. I said they were for Gordon knowing that I was going to eat them. Ugh. I did eat when everyone was gone. Now I'm tired and going to bed too full.

As my next journal entry demonstrates, even during food induced insomnia I was fantasizing about treats and what I might get into next. Is that sick or what?

<u>November 15, 2005 2:45 a.m.</u>

Here I am lying awake, stomach churning from eating too much too late, and thinking about the mint chocolate balls I saw on sale at the grocery store yesterday. Am I sick or what? I might as well read and write in the light rather than toss and turn in the dark.

I just read Ether 12 (*Book of Mormon*). Of course I remember the classic verse 27 which first impressed me in my college days in Lethbridge thirty years ago. I remember reading it in the old mobile home I shared with my roommates. Now here I am struggling with the same weakness and addiction I had then—food.

I'm baffled by how powerful and cunning my addiction is, especially sugar. Please Lord; make this weakness become strength to me.

As to my strength I am weak, but in thy strength I can do all things. I would like to have the strength against sugar that I have against alcohol, tobacco, caffeine, and all the other physical crutches of the world. I would like to know that sugar will not be a temptation any more than alcohol and tobacco are, that I could have the confidence in knowing I won't indulge in it no matter where I am just as I know I'll never indulge when offered coffee or tea or alcohol. Help me God.

Having lived a childhood lifestyle free of alcohol, caffeine, and tobacco, these substances never called to me. I wish that I had also lived a childhood free of sugar. Damn my parents! They should have been more strict!

# Sugar wars

It was time again for serious reflection on the pros and cons of abstinence from sugar. I was desperately trying to talk myself into the fact that life really would be better without sugar than with sugar. Alas, it did not work despite my best reasoning efforts.

November 15, 2005

9:30 p.m. I'm very tired from lying awake last night and feeling icky and overdosed on sugar again.

Here's a list of pros and cons of eating sugar.

Pros of going sugar free

- Flatus
- Weight
- Energy
- Happiness
- Youthfulness
- Better complexion
- Migraines

Cons of going sugar free

- How do I survive special occasions?
- Bad effects of sugar: moody, depressed, gassy, fat, icky, lower confidence, headaches, acne, fatigue,

yeast infections. It's really a no-brainer decision, so why am I struggling so badly right now?
- The combination of sleep deprivation and doing things that made me feel guilty (in this case, gossiping) automatically sent me into a frenzy of eating junk.

November 16, 2005 9:40 p.m.

I had a call from the hospital at 2:45 a.m. asking me to come in then and work the whole day. I declined and did my scheduled day, but I couldn't get back to sleep after the call. I was so exhausted all day and my uniform pants are getting tight again. Ugh, I feel blah and ugly and back to self-loathing.

I went to the food addiction meeting. I felt uplifted at the meeting and ready to recommit to abstinence and work the twelve-step program seriously. Then I went to pick up Gordon, gossiped some and felt guilty for it, then came home and ate a bunch of chocolate chips. Ugh. I wish I hadn't gossiped. I really do.

# Dayonedayonedayonedayone....

How many day ones can a person have? I can't even count the number of starter days I have had for dieting. These next entries are peppered with quotes from twelve-step literature alternating with pleading prayers to God. The solution had to be spiritual and I prayed in earnest for it.

<u>November 17, 2005 Day one again.</u>

Just for today I will yield to God. I will not eat sugar just for today.

"Before our hearts and lives can change, we must be willing to change our level of effort—we must become willing to go to any length."

I am willing to go to any length, even give up chocolate and sugar, to change, to beat my food addiction.

"When the pain of the problem gets worse than the pain of the solution, we'll be ready to change." Lord, I am ready. I can no longer take the emotional, physical, and spiritual pain of excess food.

I have tried my share of carnal solutions to a spiritual problem. I've spent hundreds of dollars, hours, and emotions on fitness programs, Weight Watchers, scales, Fit for Life, Weigh Down, starving, elderberry fasts... Dear God, I am ready for thy help and thou alone hast the power to change me. Please change my nature. I am ready.

My excesses only moved to other areas of my life. I now started a PhD program, adding that to my already full life. I really don't know why. It seemed that I just woke up one morning and decided to get a PhD. Not only did I have difficulty with food boundaries, I also had difficulty with other boundaries, like how much can a person reasonably cope with and still remain balanced? Speaking of balance, it doesn't seem to ever have been a part of my life. It appears that I lived in extremes of many sorts.

December 7, 2005

I had quite a pity party and sobbing spree because of two personal experiences of criticism from others. SHOT DOWN!
But I didn't crawl into the fridge or the cupboard and eat myself out. Praise the Lord for that small miracle. I managed through the grace of God to stay sober from my sugar addiction.

December 11, 2005

I've now had 24 days of sobriety from sugar addiction. Thank you Lord for removing the desire from me. I haven't even had to white-knuckle it. Praise God from whom all blessings flow. Thank you for the gift of removing my desire for sugar.

December 16, 2005

I worked an eight hour night shift in ER. UGH! But with the strength of God I made it through. Last night at work I was surrounded by cakes, cookies, chocolate, and others indulging. Not one of these items even appealed to me. Thank thee Lord for thy power to remove the desire from my body and mind to indulge in such spiritually destructive food.

This is day thirty of abstinence for me. I am feeling (despite having worked a night shift) very good—optimistic, hopeful, light, and happy.

December 17, 2005 9:30 p.m. Day 31

Thank thee Lord for carrying me through two night shifts without me succumbing to the myriad of treats at the hospital. There was poppycock, cookies, squares, chocolate, and cake.

I miraculously made it through the 2005 Christmas season without sugar, although I did rely heavily on sugar substitutes. I did however have a supply of holiday goodies in the house for my children and whoever else came and went, including my daughter's pug, though not intentionally so.

We had a lot in common, Sparky (the pug) and me. We were both short, pudgy, loved to eat and to walk. He walked many hills and valleys and miles with me. He also got into the holiday candy one night when he managed to get up on the table where treats were left. When we found him the next morning looking fat and miserable beside the empty chocolate containers, his look said it all. "I can't believe I ate the whole thing." I knew that look. I had had it many times. Just like me, as soon as Sparky was feeling better later in the day he was scratching and whining and clawing to get at more chocolate. Kindred binge spirits for sure. Been there, done that many many times over. Am I smarter than a pug?

# Nothing new under the cellulite except a new year

So now 2006 was well on its way and I was still my optimistic obsessed self. My next entry mentions winter weight gain and my desire to lose weight. Winter continued to be the time that weight piled on.

January 30, 2006

I made a measured food plan today and stuck with it except for adding a skim milk, sugar free banana/raspberry smoothie. I feel good. I want to get ten pounds off by the end of February. I feel good about getting sugar out of my life. Now I need to work on portion sizes to drop the weight I have once again added through the winter. What is it with winter and weight gain?

January 31, 2006

My food for thought today is valuing my body more than food. I don't have to be the garbage can for everyone's leftovers, using the excuse that I don't want to waste food. My body and health are of greater value than the food.

It seems that even in my sleep I did not have reprieve from my food misery.

February 1, 2006

I dreamed last night that I was stuffing myself with candy then felt very sorrowful, wondering why I would be doing that again when I was so well on my way to no sugar. Thankfully it was a dream and I can carry on with my sugarless lifestyle, or at least refined sugarless lifestyle. I have to acknowledge that I have eaten some things that contained sugar, some canned corn and crackers that had it, but this has been extremely limited.

February 5, 2006

In His strength I can do all things, even move mountains. What are the mountains in my life? Addictions, fat? Thighs?

February 8, 2006 Wt. 152.4

I had a good day with food yesterday. I've been emailing a daily food plan to a friend in the morning. It is another good exercise in awareness. It seems that each tool of the twelve-step program that I add to my plan helps in its own way. At first I thought it was silly but now I see the value of it, simply that it works. I like having a plan.

If nothing changes nothing changes, so I have been making some little changes and they really help bring about bigger changes.

February 19, 2006 Wt. 149.6

I finally dipped below 150 pounds for the first time in months.

February 27, 2006 3:00 a.m.

Why am I awake? I've been lying awake for two hours now. And it's the pits knowing that I have a twelve hour shift to do at the hospital. Why am I lying awake? Could it be the peanut butter and honey sandwich I had just before going to bed? What was I thinking? Will I ever learn or am I doomed to repeating stupid behaviors for the rest of my life? Remember this next time you want a bedtime snack.

As the next entry indicates, I felt a greater urge to eat when feeling regret and guilt over past experiences. Mothering seemed to be the biggest guilt trip for me. I felt so inadequate and alone as a single parent. Just the thought of it makes me want to dive into some ice-cream as I write.

Can I accept that I did the best with what I knew then? Recovery work counsels not to judge past behavior against current knowledge. I seem to excel at that and remind myself that I did what I could at the time. Intellectually I can do that, but emotionally I still struggle with the regrets of imperfection.

March 1, 2006

I walked to the food addiction meeting with my neighbor. While discussing parenting I suddenly wanted a peanut butter and honey sandwich. I feel very guilty and inadequate when parenting and discipline is brought up.

## March 11, 2006

Beautiful sunny day and I'm extremely grateful to God that I'm not craving excess food. What a blessing it is to have that compulsive drive gone and desire gone to overeat. Praise God from whom all blessings flow.

That short-lived praise above quickly gave way to misery again.

# The perfect food storm

At this point my professional responsibilities took a turn for the worse. As a nursing instructor I was required to drive a seventy mile distance to supervise students in a neighboring city hospital for long ten hour days. The long work days required that I was up at 3 a.m. and gone for the day for three days each week. The long days were physically and emotionally tormenting, wreaking havoc with my sleep, my mood, and my food habits. Add to that the stress of two teens off for two weeks of spring break. Fatigue, stress, anxiety—the perfect food storm!

March 14, 2006 5:30 a.m.

Yesterday by the time I got home I was very exhausted and very hungry (I had not eaten much during the day). While I made supper for my family, I ate three pieces of bread with honey, and then I ate some leftover lasagna. I continued to feel guilty and very exhausted and got into the feeling overwhelmed and catastrophic thinking mode.

Both children had friends over and I didn't want to go to bed as long as they were there so I flopped in front of the TV and watched the 24 hour news over and over again while eating popcorn and coming in and out of sleep, taking walks through the house to check on the kids. About 10:30 p.m. I told the friends it was time to go home. I fell into bed exhausted, disgusted with myself, and bloated. So besides feeling tired, guilty, frightened, I was now bloated. I'm bloated and stuffed from last night. I'm worried about what Gordon and Alicia are going to do all of spring break.

As the fatigue and food demons mounted, I desperately searched for positive affirmations in my life.

March 27, 2006 4:45 a.m.

I'm thankful that I'm not fifty pounds overweight. I'm thankful for a well-functioning body and the fitness level I've obtained through hill walking these past two years of living here.

The positive affirmations proved no match for the emotional and physical exhaustion of the long torturous work days. In retrospect I wonder why I agreed to such a set up with no mileage compensation and no accommodation compensation either. That was consistent with my people-pleasing passive nature. I assumed I had to do whatever was expected and not to advocate in any way for myself. I ate instead.

I admit it's an unhealthy pattern and one that still plagues me but less so than then. Through the weeks of that gruelling schedule, I saw myself degenerate and descend rapidly into daily eating binges and self-loathing, seemingly incapable of dealing effectively with the challenge.

March 31, 2006

I feel kind of low in confidence this morning, a bit sad, a bit scared, a bit guilty, and annoyed with myself.

Yesterday I made flax muffins: high protein, low carb, sugar free, and wheat free. The muffins are delicious and I ate several last night. I was in one of those very low energy apathetic moods and should have just gone to bed instead of flopping in front of the TV. Ugh! I felt low for the evening and ate. This reminded me that the ugly monster of overeating can very easily still rear its ugly head. Will I ever learn?

So, here I am this morning feeling all the old doubts and allowing myself to feel overwhelmed with my responsibilities, family, money, work, school etc.

April 4, 2006 3:30 a.m.

The time should indicate something. Here I am getting ready for my second torturous day of the week. Last night after getting home from work I made potato soup and went into total spiritual and emotional meltdown. I ate several pieces of bread and honey and bread and cheese (my ultimate comfort food). I knew that I was seeking comfort in food and misusing it.

That tail spun me into self-loathing and worrying over everything I perceive wrong in my life. I really hate getting into this tailspin that sleep deprivation sends me into.

April 7, 2006

I struggled very much to keep from overeating. The urge was very strong most of today. I wanted very badly to binge. When I got home, I went straight to a hot bath to avoid the kitchen, and now I'm going to bed.

## April 20, 2006

I am grateful to be reminded of the misery of overeating; now experiencing the after effects of excess pizza yesterday.

From pizza to pita, I continued to swing back and forth and up and down, but mostly up on the scale and down in mood, bringing back the guilt and grief over divorce and family failure. After all, had I not heard many times the idiom that no other success can compensate for failure in the home? I felt acutely that I had failed in my home because of divorce.

# No amount of food can compensate for failure to love myself

The grief of divorce and its subsequent loss of the family I thought I had came in waves of debilitating sadness that hit me when least expected. Like my weight problems, every time I thought I had it conquered, it returned again with even greater fury.

> May 2, 2006
>
> I have once again been knocked flat with sadness and fear. I don't know why these feelings surface now and then. Is it my period? Is it the food I've been eating? I don't know, but sometimes I feel racked with doubt, fear, and sadness.

Even after the work contract that proved to be so spiritually and emotionally destructive ended, I couldn't seem to get it back together again, back to that elusive place of balance and self-respect where I so wanted to be. I was spiralling rapidly down into that dark abyss lined with chips and chocolate and pizza, sucking me in with the illusion that comfort and love and peace would be found there.

## May 8, 2006

I find myself these past few weeks descending once again into food hell and I'm trying to understand the anatomy of this descent. I have gone from so much food control success to plummeting again into gluttony, self-loathing, doubt, fear, and sadness. What happened to me? I started to unravel when I was driving to Cranbrook three days a week during March and part of April. The fatigue was totally destructive spiritually, but I don't seem to have got out of it yet. Some days have been better than others, but I still persist in the vicious cycle of fear, worry, and guilt. In between all of this I'm eating to cover the unpleasant feelings. This only exacerbates the self-loathing.

I was clearly trapped in the self-loathing cycle of living the miseries of the past and worrying about the future while missing out on the moment. At the time only exercise seemed to shake me out of the food funks I got myself into. If I could just walk enough, I reasoned, I could walk away from the misery.

## May 16, 2006

I went for two walks and followed a food plan. I'm back on a daily food plan emailing to friends. I am getting serious again about food control. No more fatigue excuses. It's time to get with the program again and remind myself that I do want to be lean and free from compulsive eating.

The plan always worked for a while then came crashing down – not in a million little pieces, but into one big piece—me. Just me and my food obsession.

May 19, 2006

I drove Gordon to Radium last night after work. It was a lovely drive, but thoughts of chips haunted me on the way up and back. I caved in when I stopped for gas and ate a bag of chips, which I didn't enjoy as much as expected.

I had a feeding frenzy around 3 p.m., mostly bread and honey.

It's rather amazing that day after day I continued to search for the answers to my problem, whether in scriptures, diets, exercise, or service. I was on a mission of sorts and despite giving up numerous food and exercise plans, I never gave up the quest and was greatly rewarded in the summer of 2006 when something again seemed to click for me.

# Romancing the diet

Okay, full disclosure now. I do know what it was that clicked. I was taking an online doctoral course and connected with a single middle aged man in the class. We shared banter back and forth and I felt attracted to him even though we had never met. I liked his mind and discovered that he would be attending the same educational colloquium that I would be in July in Phoenix Arizona. And THAT was what clicked. I couldn't bear the thought of meeting him face to face for the first time and having double chins and thighs and all that fat. I admit it! Once again I was motivated by the attention of a man and that is the fat truth.

June 13, 2006

I really am a morning person. I love the feeling of waking up light and energetic and hopeful for my life.

June 19, 2006

I had a walk around noon. I love the feel of my muscular legs and butt. I'm dropping fat again—good. I feel blessed that God has removed the desire for overeating.

June 21, 2006

I worked night shift again last night. Three nights in a row and I am grateful to God for supporting me through them without caving into food excess.

July 22, 2006

While working with a colleague, he commented on my weight loss and asked me why I've lost so much weight.

"I go to a support group for food addicts. I admitted I was powerless over food addiction and that a Higher Power could deliver me."

"You're Higher Power is doing a very good job," he said.

"God always does," I responded.

July 24, 2006

I feel so slim right now. I seem to be on a super fat-burning, low appetite mode. I'm down to 143 pounds and feel ultra-thin. I had dinner with friends. They were asking about my weight loss secrets so I told them. I love the feeling of food hell being gone.

July 25, 2006

This morning I am reading the account of Alma the Younger's (*Book of Mormon*) repentance. I love the phraseology he uses and feel that it expressed my own personal journey in many ways. I too was in the gall of bitterness and misery and in bondage to this bitterness. I too feel that I have been rescued from this pit of pride and bitterness and liberated to enjoy soul freedom. It's a great way to be. Some may think that sugar abstinence is great denial, but in fact it has given me tremendous growth and joy. I'm not suffering by denying myself excess food. I am rewarding and liberating myself.

In August my youngest daughter and I went on a trail ride vacation. This next entry occurred while on that vacation camping in the Porcupine Hills of Southern Alberta.

<u>August 15, 2006</u>

I rode about six hours yesterday. Stormy, my horse, and I are kindred spirits. I had a good day herding cattle. My blue jeans are wonderfully loose, more so than the last time I wore them.

<u>August 27, 2006</u>

Dear God,

Every time I try on my small size clothes and look in the mirror I am thankful for Thy bounteous mercy in delivering me from food addiction.

Delivery from food addiction never seemed to be a once and done type of thing. I was never sure why that was. Had I not exercised (literally!) enough faith? Had I not admitted in enough ways and means and languages that I was powerless over food? What lacked I yet?

# To eat is human, to overeat is more human

As seasons passed so did my wonderful magical high of weight loss (that and I never did see the man again.). The beginnings of the end started showing in these coming entries. At this time I was finished with the full time work at the college and living on casual shift work at the hospital. It was always unpredictable whether there would be enough work week to week. Although there were nursing jobs available, I opted to not pursue them in an effort to avoid chronic shift work and body fluids.

Uncertainty about income and certainty about family needs and expenses made for the worry that left me wallowing in food.

> September 18, 2006
>
> I went to Calgary on Thursday to take Alicia for dental surgery. It was uneventful except for driving through a blizzard in the Longview area. As soon as I saw the snow I wanted to eat and have been struggling this past week with eating more than needed.
>
> September 20, 2006
>
> I ate too much after work, grilled cheese sandwiches and then bread and honey.

I went to a twelve-step meeting tonight and needed to refocus on overcoming my addiction.

September 22, 2006

I feel so much better waking after an evening of food abstinence. Help me remember this wonderful feeling that abstinence brings.

Yesterday I worked again in ER. After work I had a short nap instead of eating my fatigue, then I made supper and went for a walk.

Besides the day to day concerns and stress of life, I began now to notice the changes in my middle-aged body that signalled I was drying up. I mean my eggs were drying up and with them my youthful hormones. I was entering menopause. Here comes another wrench thrown into my life plans and food plans and whatever else plans.

September 25, 2006

I think my body is trying to menopause. I woke up about 3:00 this morning, sweaty and hot with the beginnings of a headache. I took off my PJ's and lay awake worrying about money again. Am I making a mistake to have not taken the full time nursing jobs? Am I making a mistake to spend so much on education? I worried about being a bad mother, etc. I pigged out, made bread, have a headache, and am now going to bed.

Sometime in 2006 spiritual health began to take precedence over financial health. I had made a decision to no longer work on Sundays. I wanted my Sundays to worship and nourish my spiritual health. This decision cost me a lot of blocks of work covering vacation relief.

While taking this leap of faith, I often worried about where it would land me. Trusting in God and His plan still didn't always leave me confident and sure of day to day financial needs being met. Would He pull through for me or not was often a nagging doubt I had. Still I exercised the trust, threw reason to the wind, and set it all out there for God to manage.

September 26, 2006

I worked again in ER. I had a food meltdown tonight and binged. I feel so exhausted and concerned about money and what I'll have as a job.

Day by day the work came and I moved forward not knowing what each day would bring except that it brought a lot of food. That was the one absolute certainty in my life. Food, blessed fattening food.

## Just say NO

It was always difficult for me to say no to my children and to almost anyone else except myself. This annoying trait has got me into many an unpleasant predicament and the fall of 2006 was no different.

My seventeen year old son wanted a dog and nagged me quite effectively for one, all the time searching online for the dog of his dreams (damn the internet anyway!). It wasn't enough that I had got him a cat and a horse a few years earlier and had built a paddock and a barn and bought hay. No! Now we had to get an infernal dog to complete his life. In all fairness, his little sister owned a pug so it was only fair that they both have a dog. And what did I have? I had food and I had diets.

Why in Heaven's name I agreed to this ridiculous plan I'll never know, but anyway we got a dog from a shelter in a neighboring town. A Rottweiler no less! I knew nothing about dogs in general and even less about this dog I was dragging home. I am the first to admit that I am clearly lacking in certain intellectual domains. Where my kids are concerned, I do almost anything for them. Shorty was the big dog we dragged home. He was a disaster waiting to happen and immediately caused tension in the neighborhood. It's no wonder I started eating uncontrollably again.

October 10, 2006

Yesterday I worked eight hours in ER. It was a quiet day. I ate my way through my 51st birthday. Then I took Shorty for a long walk after work while my children had Thanksgiving dinner with their dad.

I did my turkey dinner on Sunday.
I overate and now I've got major digestive flatulence. Ugh. I must get ready for the day of work.

October 11, 2006

Here I am descending into food hell once again. Ugh. What's wrong with me? Why can't I stop this ugly habit? Why is it when I feel insecure and doubting that I turn to overeating? I don't want to gain weight again. I love being lean and I want to stay lean.

October 12, 2006

For this week, I have a local twelve-step sponsor and I'm going to phone her every day. I need to refocus on the tools for overcoming addiction. Telephoning is one that I haven't used. I phoned her this morning to commit to a good day. I did eat four chocolate cookies this evening when watching a movie with Joan and Alicia.

The glory slim days of summer gave way to the overeating days of fall and on to the fat days of winter.

October 17, 2006

Yesterday I had the most ferocious migraine with nausea and vomiting. I suffered badly in the afternoon and evening. I'm not sure what precipitated it except maybe some bad eating. I am starting to let sugar creep back into my diet. I've gotta stop that again. I haven't had such a bad migraine in over a year.

What's odd about my behavior is that yesterday while in the throes of my migraines and nausea I could not imagine ever eating again, especially what may have been the offending food. Today of course, as soon as I feel better I'm struggling to focus again on not overindulging. I certainly don't want to feel sick all the time to avoid eating.

October 26, 2006

I'm exhausted and I'm on another food bender. How did I get to this state again? I am self-loathing, pigging out, not caring about myself. I've got to get off sugar again. I know it's destructive to me.

October 27, 2006

What's this obsession I have with food? I'm sick. I'm back into stinky sugar thinking, convincing myself that I have to have sugar to enjoy life when in fact it is life without sugar and excess food that is really enjoyable.

October 30, 2006

Today I start anew on the sugar free journey. I know that my irritability, loss of appetite control, and pride are influenced by sugar addiction.

November 7, 2006

What's wrong with me? I'm slipping back into food hell. My house is a mess. I'm either at work, asleep, travelling to volleyball tournaments, or working on my doctoral courses.

I feel at loose ends and restless. I'm eating myself into oblivion to avoid thinking and feeling.

The tension and dog days of Shorty escalated with his attack on a neighbor's dog. I had to deal with it in a more effective way than eating, avoidance, and denial. So one weekend when both my teens were away playing volleyball, I took him to the vet and paid to have him put to sleep. I bawled like a baby sitting in the vet's office with the dog's head on my knee waiting for his demise to take place. He died. I ate. The combined vet bill from the dog he attacked and putting him to sleep resulted in a huge bill that flipped me into my insecurity cycle where I worried and ate and worried and ate.

November 19, 2006

I'm feeling blah this evening. My weight is going up again and I'm feeling out of control. I'm trying to write off my funk.

Writing myself slim didn't work then, nor does it now.

## She that loses her fat shall find it

The dog was gone. Too bad my feeding frenzy didn't go with him. Too bad I couldn't just put my food monster to sleep with the same simple injection that put my dog to sleep. But alas, it was not that simple. My weakness persisted, dog or not, and my daily spiritual pursuits still likened all scripture to my problem.

November 26, 2006

I had turkey dinner at friends. I ate too much pumpkin pie and some chocolate cake and now I feel stuffed. I'm feeling insecure again over my finances and insecure about school and the cost and wondering if it was a big mistake to invest so much into education.

November 27, 2006

It's a stormy, windy, snowy morning. I had an unsettled sleep with restless dreams and fear, probably precipitated by my excess food last night. I really loathe lying awake feeling fear and regret and feeling like I wish I hadn't started this PhD program. It has set me back financially and I'm feeling overwhelmed with it.
Now I must try to nurture myself without excess food.

November 28, 2006

Unfortunately I had a pig-out evening last night, but today is another day and I'm going to be abstinent today.

December 4, 2006

I ate myself through the stress of the week, being around my ex-husband at the volleyball tournament everyday. I am reminded of my failure as a wife and I'm thinking that's what is so uncomfortable about being around him. Add to that the Christmas season and this compounds my feelings of failure with sadness and grief for the loss of my home and security as it was in Lister. Add to that my anxieties over money and my weakness for spending to excess for my children. Then there's the guilt over spending money on my education rather than on them for Christmas. So I ate myself through the week and now I suffer once again. But today is a new day and I have recommitted myself to abstinence just for today.

8:30 p.m. I was okay until after supper then I ate myself through the evening very aware that I have a big addiction. What's wrong with me? I feel like I am intentionally getting fat again because that's where I belong. Help me stop.

# Eat it and it will go away

I am convinced that my annoying character trait of ignoring things rather than addressing them has contributed to much of my compulsive overeating. Somewhere inside me I have not had the courage to advocate for myself, to ask for needed help. Instead of dealing with money issues, I ate. It is obvious in these entries filled with concern over money and yet I was not able to ask for the legally mandated financial assistance expected from my ex-spouse. This caused only further frustration and self-loathing for being so gutless and timid.

I read somewhere that we teach people how to treat us and if we act like doormats, we will be walked on. I knew that I was a doormat and had been for quite some time. This only compounded my self-loathing. I knew that I had taught people how to treat me. I had played the doormat role and could not get out of it after so many years of being walked on. Eating kept me down in my comfortable fat doormat role.

December 5, 2006

I am feeling blue again and eating again. I am feeling down, scared, sad, mourning for my secure home of the past, and wishing for things to be different.

December 6, 2006

I've had a wonderfully abstinent day: no compulsive eating, no sugar, no refined carbohydrates, no junk food, just decent whole food in moderation and I feel so hopeful and happy.

December 7, 2006

I am grateful for another abstinent day. I am so much happier when I don't eat sugar and junk food and when I eat in moderation. Help me remember this Lord, next time I am tempted to pig out.

The wonderful warm fuzzy feeling of all is well ended abruptly with the presence of goodies at work.

December 11, 2006

Anatomy of a binge: I woke up feeling great and ate my breakfast of power—yogurt with ground flax and fruit and a handful of almonds.
I got to work and saw a plate of dates with filling. I tried one thinking it was just dates and walnuts. It turned out to have a delicious caramel sweet filling and I was hooked. Ugh. I pigged out after work then went to a volleyball party at a friend's. I had to take a treat, so I bought Nanaimo bars. Ugh, more food. Now I feel like crap again.

December 14, 2006

I am having a fruit day today to flush out the junk of the week. I didn't sleep well. The past few nights I woke up at 3:00 a.m. and my mind churns for the rest of the night.

December 17, 2006

I went snowboarding yesterday. After four runs I felt very dizzy and nauseated with a migraine coming on so I spent the day huddled in the lodge sick. Ugh. I know it was from food excess the day before. There I was, once again suffering because of allowing excess food to destroy my health.
Got home about 6:30 p.m., had a hot bath, and went to sleep. Ugh!
So now let December 16th be the start of abstinence from sugar and junk food. Why has it taken me so much pain to remember the effects of junk food and excess? Am I not a very slow learner?

December 20, 2006

I feel so much better when I abstain from overeating, especially abstaining from junk and sugar. I sleep better. I awake feeling peaceful. Life is simply much better. Remember, remember, remember.

The memory ended with the coming of another Christmas Season.

# Deck the thighs with tons of turtles

Should old addictions be forgot and never brought to mind? I don't think so. As the last week of the year drew nigh, I was deeply entrenched once again in the throes of food addiction.

December 25, 2006

I worked a twelve hour day in ER—the worst binge day I've had in years. I pigged out on sweets and junk all day and I feel absolutely rotten. Hopefully it is my last food binge. I'm abstaining right now and plan to get sugar out of my life once again.

December 26, 2006

I've had a good sleep and am grateful to God for that. It is in a good night sleep that I can feel refreshed and ready to face a positive day of abstinence.

Just for today I will abstain from all processed foods. Just for today I will eat whole fresh fruit and vegetables.

December 30, 2006

I feel so much better when I don't eat junk and excess. Please help me remember minute by minute how much better I feel not to overeat and not to eat refined foods.

Here I go again with my predictable goal setting session as another year comes around. So far all I had done was recycle myself in and out of being fat then less fat, then fat, then more fat. The one constant in my life was my indestructible hope that someday I would conquer once and for all.

2007 Goals:

- Abstain from all refined and processed foods i.e. sugar, white flour, rice, and hydrogenated oils.
- No clothing purchases until I weigh 130 pounds

As per usual, the first day of the year was a fast of some sort, intending to 'shock' my system into not liking to eat. Reeeeeeeeaaaally!?

January 1, 2007

I had a fruit day and I feel better already. I don't like descending into food hell. I want to recapture the serenity of abstinence.

January 9, 2007

I am thankful for a week of abstinence from sugar and junk food and subsequently compulsive eating. What a good week I have been blessed with. Serenity increases as sugar decreases—I guess I could say there is a negative correlation there. I just started my advanced stats course.

January 21, 2007

Twenty-one days into the new year and I've been blessed with abstinence from sugar and junk food. I feel good about that.

# My fridge through troubled water

In late January my teenage son was suspended from school for an after school fight. I was very distraught and used the only weapon I felt comfortable with: writing, that and eating.

February 1, 2007

I have felt for most of my life that I had no voice. I don't like that feeling. I think that's why I like writing so much. It's where I find my voice and express it.
I feel intimidated by authority and often my mind goes blank and I don't think to challenge the claims that are made.
It's a terrible feeling to be intimidated and have your voice squelched out of fear. That's when I eat. I fear speaking my mind because I might be wrong and look like an idiot.
I fear the prideful monster that lives within. I fear deceit and humiliation. I fear obesity. I fear the food monster that lies beneath and wants to destroy my eternal soul with greed and excess. I fear my insecurities. I guess I fear living my truth at all times so I revert to another truth to protect the insecurities I have. I think I need to talk to Freud.
NO. I need to talk with God.

And talk to God I have done, over and over and over again. Perhaps what I need more is to listen to God rather than talk to God. I read a quotation that when you do all the talking, you only learn what you already know. It certainly seemed that way for me, going through a revolving door of dieting and binging. In the next entry I am trying to remind myself who it is I worship and who it is that I am. Somehow that reminder had to occur over and over again.

<u>February 2, 2007</u>

Each time I am tempted I will remind myself of my identity. What is food that I should worship it?

I'm so mad at myself for gaining weight again. Here I am back up to 150 pounds. I was probably 160 at the New Year. In the fall I was down to 143 and feeling great. Now I've got rolls again around my middle and I hate the feeling. Why, why, why did I let the feeding monster out again? I love being thin and feeling light and energetic, but once I get into sugar I'm on a feeding rampage that quickly fills out my fat cells again. Ugh!

# The food Ferris wheel

Between worship and visualization and dieting and binging and life stresses thrown into the mix, I was still a cacophony of emotions battling to be heard and seen and loved. From peace and joy to turmoil and despair, it's all recorded over and over again in the journals of my life.

February 25, 2007

I just got in from my morning walk. I feel happy, hopeful, peaceful, optimistic, intelligent, and loved. Is this not the ultimate abundance?

This is my ultimate visualization for what I want: physical health, youth, fitness, leanness—130 pounds of energy, beauty, and vitality.

March 4, 2007

I feel so much more peace in my life without sugar and junk food. I'm so thankful to be free from that addiction these past two months. What a tremendous spiritual blessing it is not to have food rule my life. Good health, energy, and vitality taste so much better than junk food or any food taken in excess.

March 12, 2007

I'm exhausted and I've eaten too much. Alicia talked me into having a barbecue for the girls' and boys' basketball teams so there was junk food that kids brought and I indulged in some chips. Ugh. I also ate hotdogs. Ugh too.

March 13, 2007

I had a fruit only day to clear my body of chips and hot dog (poison).

April 3, 2007

Yesterday I felt sad, anxious, and overwhelmed. I am not sure why but I definitely used food to feed my spiritual and emotional hunger.
Finally about 8 p.m. I stopped my eating and started cleaning. Part of my downer was looking at how grungy my house is. I cleaned out a closet, did some vacuuming, cleaned the kitchen, and then went to bed.

April 5, 2007

I went to my food addiction meeting last night and feel uplifted and hopeful this morning. The desire to abstain from compulsive eating is renewed and I feel more hopeful than I have these past few days.

I seemed so adept at writing lists of what I wanted to be and visualizing what I wanted in my life. The only problem was that the list and vision never quite materialized. So much for *the secret* in my life.

## April 11, 2007

I feel poisoned having had pizza and sugar free ice-cream (way too much) last night. It's time to commit myself to abstinence from overeating. I need to be abstinent from:

1. sugar and all its substitutes
2. white flour—all refined carbs
3. bread very sparingly
4. salt
5. all food after 5 p.m.

I've been overeating the past week and sleeping poorly—excess gas, agitated, anxious, and tense.

This is my body visual: I want to weigh 130 pounds.

If only I could never have had any stress in my life I may have been able to keep it all together and live a balanced life. At least, that's what I tried telling myself.

## Son of a binge!

My youngest was now entering that dreaded puberty stage where kids lose their brains, hate their moms, and think they know everything. I was grieving the loss of my last child to hormones and wasn't prepared for her changing personality. She was in puberty while I was in reverse puberty. It didn't help that I had all this self-induced anxiety by insisting on taking expensive doctoral level courses despite insufficient funds. What was I thinking? Oh ya, I wasn't—I was in reverse puberty. My mind may have been gone, but my appetite sure the hell wasn't.

April 13, 2007

I ate too much again last night. I know part of my restless eating is some anxiety over the course that started this week but I haven't been able to start it because I haven't yet paid for it.
I am also experiencing some anxiety over my daughter and I am having some inner conflict.

April 14, 2007

I know that God cares about my life. He cares what I eat, what I look like, how I feel who I have as friends, and what I say because all of these details contribute to what will be my eternal soul. All of these small and simple things will become my eternal soul. It **does** matter what I eat, what I drink, what I say, what I think, what I read, what I listen to, who I spend time with, and where I spend time.

### April 15, 2007

I just want to walk peaceably with people and I want to weigh 130 pounds.

Here comes some more positive self-talk and affirmations. You'd think by now I had practically affirmed myself into a coma. Yet I was still eating after all these affirmations.

### April 16, 2007

Just for today I will trust in abstinence from sugar, from refined carbs, from junk food, and from compulsive overeating.
I want optimum health. I want to respect my body for the magnificent creation that it is. I want to weigh 130 pounds. I want to love and honor this temple of my spirit.

### April 17, 2007

I had a moderate feeding frenzy of left over chicken fingers then bread and honey. Not sure why.

### April 19, 2007

Just for today I will abstain from excess eating. I will eat only in response to hunger and in amounts to satisfy the hunger (physical hunger, not emotional hunger).
Just for today I will remember my goal of health and beauty. I will love and cherish my body. I want to be

free from compulsive eating. I want peace with the temple of my spirit.

10:00 p.m. Ugh. I went to a women's church group meeting, which was an ethnic potluck, and I overate. I feel stuffed and gross and lonely and all those things I don't want to feel. What a binge! I want to be abstinent from this compulsion. I want to be lean and healthy and free from those chaotic icky feelings of being out of control. I want to weigh 130 pounds. I want beauty and strength.

April 20, 2007 6:30 a.m.

Ugh. I feel so poisoned this morning having used food as a drug last night. I feel sorry for my poor body.

8:30 a.m. I just had a good hike with some friends. I am suffering the effects of excess food from last night.

April 25, 2007

I went to an addiction meeting tonight and I feel so much more hopeful and positive than I've felt giving into food these past weeks.
I desperately needed help to get me out of the negative food binging cycle I was in. I am thankful for the meeting.

April 26, 2007

I feel so much more hopeful today and focused on wanting God in my life.

9:00 p.m. I've had a wonderful abstinent day and my whole outlook on life has gone back to being hopeful, optimistic, and trusting in God. I'm happy again after such a turbulent and unsettled few weeks.

<u>April 27, 2007</u>

All things are becoming spiritual to me as the Lord intended. The more spiritual food I ingest, the less carnal food I need.

Nothing could prepare me for the tragic shock that was about to hit my family.

# Earth has no sorrow that Heaven cannot heal

On April 29, 2007 my nineteen year old nephew committed suicide, sending the whole family into an emotional melt down. Sorrow and regret and anger enveloped us all for months to come. The emotional turbulence sent me quickly spinning into an extended feeding frenzy.

June 26, 2007

Where do I begin? I am once again back in the Babylonian binge mode with sugar on my mind and hips and butt. I am reminded of the scripture that talks of the dog returning to its vomit and the sow to her wallowing in the mud. I'm the sow returning to my wallowing in food hell.

June 27, 2007

I am reading Helaman chapters 12 & 13 (*Book of Mornon*). I am likening it to my carnal eating hell. When I get into my eating frenzy and let junk food and sugar rule my life I feel the disconnect from the Spirit and I start allowing myself to be ruled by pride and vain things. I become inconsiderate, gossipy, sarcastic—all these worldly things that I don't want to be. Just for today I will abstain from sugar and refined carbohydrates.

Old doubts returned about money and the choice I made to get a PhD. The stress continued. It didn't help that I worked only temporary contracts rather than taking a full time permanent position in nursing.

It's strange that no matter how bad money situations get, there's still money for overeating. Why is that, I wonder? I hear it's the same for smoking and drinking habits. Booze sales seem to flourish no matter how bad the economy gets and I know of many smokers who clearly can't afford to smoke. I guess food is my addiction for hard times. The harder the times, the more food I seemed to eat.

July 3, 2007

I feel apathetic, desperate, anxious, overwhelmed, and wishing I had never started a PhD. I wouldn't be in the financial bind I find myself in right now.
I'm eating and struggling and eating and struggling and I think I'm going through menopause now and I'm gaining weight, worrying about money, and craving sweets.

July 7, 2011

Once again I have focused on God and been lifted from the hell of food obsession. There is definitely a very, very negative impact of sugar on me. When I start eating sugar and any refined carbohydrates or junk food I descend into a whirlpool of depression, pessimism, self-loathing, and fear. It's a bad place to be.

## July 15, 2007

I've been walking and eating a lot. I am back to my sugar cottage in Babylon. I find the hospital work environment a difficult place to maintain abstinence and I must rally greater strength to get back to a positive eating plan. I have also missed several food addiction meetings because some of the food group people are away and the core group has not been available.

# Check bounced, diet bounced

July 19, 2007

I had a phone message that the check I wrote for strawberries bounced. Ugh. I quickly got cash and made restitution. What a pain that is. I cried, feeling low and lonely, but I did not turn to food even though there was pizza on the kitchen counter.

July 22, 2007

What a blessing it is to awaken to fasting, knowing that I have not given in to food addiction for four days. I've had four glorious days of no junk food and no sugar.
My body, mind, and spirit are so much happier and peaceful when I avoid refined carbs.

July 25, 2007

I'm grateful to have had abstinence from sugar and junk and overeating again now for the past week. What a tremendous blessing it is. I'm so grateful that once again Christ has pulled my sorry butt out of the food hell into which I had descended. I feel an infusion of hope, joy, and peace again and I feel the momentum of abstinence. Please help me stay on this strait but hopeful and joy-filled course.

August 11, 2007

Last night I went out for a long bike ride, about 25 kilometres. It was the first bike ride I've done in two years. I biked all the way up Beam Road. In the night my knees were throbbing but I got up this morning, took some Advil, and went out for a walk. I love feeling fit.

I have eaten so many cherries my belly is boiling and I've got diarrhea. Some orchardist friends have been giving us cherries—delicious cherries! I've been pigging out on them every day.

My third child, Gordon, graduated high school and spent the summer preparing to move away to university on a volleyball scholarship. His intended university held volleyball camps in the local high school. My son helped with the camp and I helped by billeting one of the university athletes. It was a simple task, but still just enough to tip me over the food edge again.

August 13, 2007

I feel exhausted and stuffed. Once again I've descended into food hell. I don't even know why. I just started eating. I guess I have some tension over yet another house guest.

I continued to seek for peace in exercise, and lots of it. If only I could exercise enough, I could balance the eating frenzies, I thought.

August 14, 2007

I had a long bike ride this evening. I estimate about 25 kilometres. The alfalfa bloom smells absolutely intoxicating.

## August 15, 2007

I had a busy day at work. I am now by myself and eating myself into a frenzy tonight. I'm not sure why but I've definitely lost focus from abstinence. Our food addiction group seems to have disintegrated for some reason. I hope we can get it back together again.
I definitely have trouble with eating when I'm tired. I should just take a nap instead of eating.

## August 18, 2007

Yesterday was Gordon's eighteenth birthday. I got an ice cream cake after work but no one was home. I thought if no one came along I'd eat the whole thing alone myself but I didn't. I am having bittersweet feelings as my child leaves home. We had pizza and the ice cream cake today. I'm too full again.

## Sometimes food IS love

Transitions continued to be difficult times for me and here comes another one: launching my third child out into the world. With each child launching, it seemed that part of my heart went along with them. Too bad it wasn't part of my thigh or belly or butt. I seemed to try to fill my empty mother heart with food. It didn't really work, but I did it anyway, over and over and over and over again. Insanity, I know.

August 20, 2007

Gordon left for Kamloops yesterday. Another child launched, so I felt a bit of melancholy for that.

August 26, 2007

Now I'm sitting on the toilet blowing off the excess of yesterday. We went to Costco and bought supplies, including a box of Fiber 1 bars which are very good. I've got to take inventory of my life again. I'm in a bad place as far as eating goes. Amazing how those old eating habits creep in and along with that, the pounds and fat. My clothes are once again snug.

10:00 p.m. I am so bloated with excess and feeling so uncomfortable. All the excess food makes me feel so miserable. What's the matter with me? Now my house is empty; it's just Alicia and me. Starting now I'm back to using the recovery tools to get back to God.

I love the feeling of moderation, of going sugar free, of eating for what my body needs. Here I go again for a more peaceful me.

Tomorrow and Tuesday I am going to do "take off" days: lean protein, green veggies, and a cantaloupe. Then I'll get back on no sugar or refined carbohydrates and no junk food. It will be a relief.

August 31, 2007

O remember, remember, remember, the joy of abstinence from sugar, from junk food, from overeating. Remember the awfulness of excess eating: flatulence, tight clothes, lethargy, ugh.

Remember the liberating feelings of love, joy, peace, beauty, and health that come with abstinence. Lord, help me to keep my appetite within the bounds that Thou hast set.

For the fall months 2007 I was employed in a community nurse position as a consultant for mentally challenged adults in the community. This was a temporary part time position to see me through the fall until my next teaching contract with the college. For a time it assuaged my concern over money and I continued to live an abstinent life filled with lots of exercise.

September 10, 2007

I had a two hour bike ride tonight.

September 22, 2007

I spent the day watching Alicia play volleyball.

I had a good hike this morning then a walk between games then another hike to the top of the church hill with my sister tonight in the dark. I had eaten four Fiber 1 bars today and wanted to walk them off.

# The revolving diet door

My older daughter was struggling with where her life was going and returned home for a time to sort out her plans. I worried and stressed over choices she was making, which was more fodder for food addiction. I felt guilty that her last year of high school was so miserable because of her parents' separation and I felt that she was struggling in her young adult years as a result of this. I felt angst and sadness and helpless to help her and just wanted to eat. And eat I did.

September 27, 2007

I've eaten too much today, mostly fiber bars. I've got to not eat them anymore. I'm bloated and gassy from consuming way too many. Gotta stop it again.

October 1, 2007

How pathetic is this? I ate five Fiber 1 bars and a chocolate bar tonight. I simply must admit that I cannot eat sugar. I'm gradually getting more and more into it again and losing spiritual focus.

I must reconfirm my goals to keep them fresh before me. I want to be lean, fit, and beautiful and down to 130 pounds by Christmas. If this is going to happen then I must follow my measured meal plan perfectly from now until then. I cannot afford to binge on sugar or bread or any other substance. If 130 pounds is the weight I want then I must be willing to pay the price.

October 3, 2007

Last night we went to a church function for youth. I ate too much and dessert too. Today I am on refocus and commitment to abstinence mode. No sugar seems to be the best mode for me. Just for today I will be abstinent from excess food and abstinent from sugar and refined carbs.

October 4, 2007

I had a pleasant work day.

I got in three hours of walking today: half an hour before work and lunch then two hours after work. I am feeling good. Increasing spirituality through fewer physical indulgences makes me feel loved, peaceful, joyful, and hopeful.

October 5, 2007

2 Nephi 9: 39 (*Book of Mormon*). Being carnally minded IS death. Excess food brings death sooner than temperance and moderation. I have been very carnally minded with food. Forgive me Lord for the destruction I have caused to this beautiful temple Thou has given me.

Even from morning meditation to night, my focus shifted so fast that I could hardly keep up with myself. Here is the end of day journaling showing the departure from the spiritual high I felt in the morning. It seemed that all I needed to do was step out of my bedroom, see food, and I was distracted like a two year old in a candy store. Those damn holidays filled with food don't help. Must I live in a monastery or on a Tibetan mountain to manage my feeding behavior?

> 9:30 p.m. I've eaten too much pumpkin pie. I had a turkey dinner here and invited the family. I cooked the turkey and everyone else brought something to go with it. Now I'm stuffed and remembering the awfulness of yielding to the enticing of that cunning one who makes carnal excess appear so pleasurable and cozy and comforting. Ah well, another day is done and I'm going to let it go as I press forward with renewed commitment to abstinence.

The blessed Thanksgiving holiday passed but the excess pumpkin pie settled in on my butt and thighs. It's a reminder, once again, that food excess is not easily forgotten or beaten.

> October 13, 2007
>
> I felt many blessings today watching Alicia play volleyball and enjoying her talent.
>
> I was also blessed to have several good walks and ate a pile of ice cream and raspberries and blueberry muffins.
>
> October 15, 2007 Worked 7a.m. - 7 p.m.
>
> I ate way too much after working hectically until almost 6 p.m. I was famished and started wolfing down food until now when I'm going to bed at 9 p.m., tired and full.
>
> October 16, 2007
>
> I woke up feeling blue and anxious and afraid about life, having eaten to excess last night, ice cream etc. My

throat hurts and my head feels plugged this morning because of it. That then leads me to negativism, fear, and pessimism.

At this time I received notice that Revenue Canada was not accepting my education expenses as deductions because I was not full time and was taking courses online from the States. I was required to pay back about $4,000. What to do? Eat! I tried desperately to talk myself out of food as a solution to financial woes. It seemed to work for only a day or two.

October 18, 2007

Eating will not make my financial problems or Revenue Canada go away.

October 23, 2007

Mondays seem to be a real blue day for me. I felt sad all day and scared and alone. I came home from work and slept and watched TV eating ice-cream and raspberries. I just had this overwhelming sad feeling all day. Sort of an insecure, money scared type of day.

# The sugary slope to hell

The next entry discloses again my long held belief that sugar in my body was a depressant, and yet I could not seem to talk myself out of this self-destructive substance. Cognitive dissonance ruled as I continued to want peace and balance and a lean body, but I also wanted to eat and I wanted to eat lots.

October 24, 2007

Sugar depresses me so why am I back into it? Let me change again, just for today. I thank God that I'm not carved in stone, that today is a new day to repent, be forgiven, and move forward without guilt. Look to God and live. Do not look to sugar or addiction or any carnal pleasure. Look to God and commit. Commit, then the power of God will lift you up as on eagle wings and carry you above carnal addictions: the power of commitment.

At this point in my education I was preparing to conduct heuristic research for my dissertation and was required to explore other heuristic studies done. Wouldn't you know I would find one dealing with food addiction? It attracted my attention as fast as any magic weight loss cure could. I intensified my efforts to work the twelve-step program by searching for an online sponsor. Our little group of food addicts seemed to be floundering and none of us felt successful enough to be sponsors.

As much as we loved each other, we just couldn't seem to get it together enough to provide the needed support. It was time to get more serious.

October 26, 2007

Thank Thee for the heuristic dissertation I found on spiritual recovery of food addiction. Thank Thee for the sponsor list I got from the online food addiction program. Thank Thee for the lovely walk. Thank Thee for abstinence from compulsive eating.

My last baby was beginning to explore her independence and hitting that dreaded phase where I was no longer the focus of her life. Now what? How could I get my own life when my life had been my children's lives for over two decades and I didn't want to give that up? I didn't want to be me; I wanted to continue being someone's mother.

October 29, 2007 6:30 a.m.

For some reason Mondays have been difficult for me these past few weeks. I'm not exactly sure why. Today I'm going to focus extra strongly on positive affirmations by looking to God to keep the day in focus spiritually as I go off to the hospital for a twelve-hour shift.

10:00 p.m. Though I'm feeling a bit blue I'm grateful to have not binged today. I feel sad.

October 30, 2007

I feel frustrated and sad and angry and gutless and a failure as a parent. All this tonight and I didn't binge. I'm lonely.

I had an email today from my online sponsor and she's going to be my sponsor for the twelve-step food addiction program.

November 1, 2007 6:45 a.m.

I admit I am powerless over junk food, sugar, refined carbohydrates, and my life as an addict is unmanageable.

I know my body is a temple and God has provided me with knowledge to beautify, strengthen, and maintain my temple. That food and life and body maintenance guide is the Word of Wisdom. (Doctrine and Covenants section 89).

I listened to the news last night and heard yet again another study supporting living God's food plan. A third of all cancer could be prevented if people lost weight—fat and junk food are killing us.

Having connected with an online sponsor, I received assignments from her and responded to her questions. Some of these responses are included in the next month's journal entries.

# Me food and Satan

The program of twelve-step work is an interesting concept. I don't think it is meant to end and I like to know that there are ends because of the admonition to endure to the end. To what end should I endure when there really is no end? It just keeps on going, twelve steps around and around and around again, not twelve weeks, but twelve steps in continual motion over and over and over again. It's sort of like my dieting years so I should have really fit right in there. My journal thoughts continue to focus heavily (damn it!) on twelve-step work.

November 2, 2007

I am willing to search deep inside to my spiritual self to conquer my carnal addiction of food. I hadn't realized the power of the word 'action' as applied to abstinence and writing, nor had I internalized these as the most personal and powerful and thus the ones that the adversary wants to discourage. I feel enlightened to have this finally click in to my head after more than two years of reading and attending food addiction meetings.

November 3, 2007

Carnally minded really is death. Excess food is an early death. Not only is it early death, it's also death by degrees as parts of the body's functioning gradually die with excess fat. Arteries clog and body areas die. Not only this, but spirituality dies, hope dies, and faith dies. Joy dies. Self-respect dies. Beauty dies. Love dies. Peace dies. Relationships die.

After decades of trying to manage my carnal self according to the intelligence of my creature self, I know that my only hope of reprieve is through the power of God. Some of my past and present habits and behaviors have made me aware that I am still capable of unleashing the pride of the feeding monster within. It may hide as if subdued for a time but seems to resurface just when I think that I have it beat.

It is these experiences with thinking I've conquered the enemy finally once and for all only to find myself buried head first in a bag of chips that make me aware that this is definitely a progressive disease. When my rationalizing starts up again arguing that treats are not sin, and after all I'm not drinking or smoking, so what's the big deal, then my peace leaves and the unsettled fears resurface as I see myself slipping away from the only Source of peace and love that has proven trustworthy in my life. No amount of food is worth that loss of spiritual security and peace.

When I go to the food compulsively, I know that I have chosen to look to it as a source of comfort when what I really need is to feel the hope and peace of the Spirit and trust that the peace it offers is far greater than that of food. When I choose God, I am always relieved; when I choose the excess food I always regret it.

It is not only the excess food I regret but the feelings of insecurity, fear, doubt, anger, jealousy, and negativity that come with it. The compulsive habit feeds the negativity and pessimism and soon I find myself being rude, sarcastic, insensitive, and generally unlovable. In short, I am worshipping carnality and hating myself doing it. Resisting the compulsion to eat leads to the peace that only God can give.

Why then would anyone in his or her right mind choose compulsive eating over abstinence? I guess that demonstrates the un-rightness of mind or insanity of anyone giving into such behavior. It really is not fun. It is torment and agony as I separate farther from God and closer to dumb idols.

Food goeth before destruction and a heavy butt before a fall

I seemed to spend a lot of time dwelling on the topic of pride certain that therein was the core of my problem as believed in addiction recovery work.

Nov 5, 2007

From a former LDS church president's talk on pride, I learned that one sign of pride is allowing appetites to go beyond the bounds that the Lord has set. Excess eating and eating those things that do not have a positive effect on the body demonstrate my will pitted against God's will. As long as I am pitting my will against His by exceeding the boundaries He has set, I cannot have a personal relationship with Him, but can only live on the fringes of knowing about Him but not knowing Him.

Another talk that has influenced my eating behavior and echoes in my mind when I feel tempted to cave into the carnal ways of junk food is a talk by an LDS apostle given before he was an apostle, "Ye are the temple of God". He states that those who know the true nature of their bodies and the role of these bodies would never knowingly put anything into their bodies that does not have a positive effect. Also mentioned in this talk is the fact that my body is not mine but is on loan from God. How can I destroy this temple that is not mine but belongs to God? Knowing this reinforces the need I have to care for the loan. Destroying this body wilfully will destroy any hope of a personal loving relationship with the owner of my body. How can I experience a loving relationship with God while at the same time destroying the temple He has loaned to me?

<u>November 6, 2007</u>

Compulsive eating is definitely a carnal problem and so have many of my 'fixes' for the problem. Diet after diet, from the extreme to the more balanced, as well as supplements promising to speed up my metabolism, I have spent a fortune in worldly solutions always looking for that diet to end all diets without getting to the core of the problem: pride, unwillingness to accept the boundaries God has set for my body, and using food for love, comfort, hate, revenge, and security.

Just now I am feeling some anxiety over a message I had to phone Gordon's volleyball coach. What could be wrong I wonder? When I returned the call I got voicemail and left a message, then I called Gordon and got voicemail, so then the first thing I turn to is food. Two pieces of whole grain bread with honey later and

I am stopping here before I descend into food hell over some anticipated problem that may or may not exist. Why am I anticipating that the call was bearing negative information? I wish I could clear it up right now rather than worry about what it might be.

Anyway, food will not fix anything but will only make me go in a tailspin to food hell and self-loathing.

Alma 26: 12 (*Book of Mormon*) I have been lured by so many worldly products promising the ultimate in assertiveness, beauty, weight loss etc. I remember an earpiece that I bought that I put into my ear for acupressure to reduce appetite. What a joke that was. Then I had those tapes that I listened to every night before sleep that were supposed to reprogram my mind into thinking thin. Then there was the money I spent on Weight Watchers, Living Light, and gym memberships, and supplements and elderberry fasts, and grapefruit fasts. They neither solved my problem nor improved my spirituality. They only made me feel worse about myself and more of a failure as I drifted farther from the Source of success and love and joy and peace.

Nov 6, 2007

The more I eat, the less I love myself and the more I hate my body. How can I hate such a marvellous creation on loan from God? How can I take the needs of my body (nourishment) and turn them into carnality through excess when all this excess is usually food (pretend food) that destroys rather than nourishes my body? It is an illusion to think that this is seeking any kind of life, but only selfish pleasure that isn't even pleasure after the first few bites. What starts as pleasure ends only in remorse, regret, fat, and headaches.

When I am seeking God's will I have only the health of my body as incentive for eating. I eat to live and glorify God through glorifying my body rather than eat to glorify a few tiny taste buds.

November 7, 2007

For many years I have known tacitly that my eating compulsion was a spiritual problem, but I had always denied how destructive it really was, and had always entertained the notion that I would magically transform sometime in the future, like January 1st of every year. It always seemed easier to pretend not to care and to speak as though those who were concerned about their appearance were the obsessed and vain ones. Pride had kept me from openly admitting that I definitely had a problem and needed Divine help to conquer it. It was much more convenient to blame my mother or genes or console myself with the lies that I was meant to be fat and that's how it would always be. Of course these soothing words never really convinced me for long, then I would be onto my next diet to end all diets, hating my friends who never seemed to gain weight but stayed the same their whole lives.

The simple act of thinking and writing reveals my true self as I know it has always been, though I tried not to know.

# The emperor's new size

I have learned over the years that most people know everyone else's problems. It is only the struggling person who pretends that no one knows and no one says anything despite the obvious being the obvious. Like the emperor's new clothes, nothing was really hidden except my head, which was buried in the sugar. Gaining weight is pretty obvious and not something you would have to be particularly astute to notice.

November 8, 2007

Just for today I can accept that I must be conscious and honest about my eating behavior. After so many years of struggling, then pretending not to care about my weight, then pretending to care, then scoffing at health fanatics, then being one, I have come to a place of transparency about who I am and how I struggle. It seems odd that I would even pretend that my eating problems have been a secret to anyone, so why try to hide them from myself? Isn't it obvious when weight goes up and down, and up and down, and up and up and then down and up again, that there is a problem? It's not like I have to inform people that the problem exists.

Struggling with the problem has not proven to be easy or enjoyable, so why should I fear honesty about it?

Certainly being honest about it as a lifetime journey cannot be worse than the struggle to conquer it by worldly temporary solutions.

There's also a shift of thought here that sees the honest and lifetime change as a blessing compared to the madness and pain of the past struggles. It's really much easier to be honest and abstinent than to deny and binge. I no longer see healthy abstinence as punishment or restriction—I see it as freedom, peace, and joy. I love the feeling of waking up with an empty stomach, clear head, optimistic anticipation for the day, and clothes that fit and look good. How could anyone think that the opposite (flatulence, bloating, sugar hangover, headaches, depression, self-loathing, tight clothes etc.) is worth any amount of any kind of food?

Can I accept the idea that this is a lifelong change? Yes. How can I possibly not choose this over the alternative tortures as mentioned above? It's like choosing eternal life over eternal death (2 Nephi 10: 23 *Book of Mormon*). Doesn't that sound like a no-brainer? Yet why would it have taken so long to clue in?

November, 2007

When does abstinence not become perfectionism? Am I not wanting perfect abstinence from the compulsion or whatever it is that triggers the compulsion?

*I came to believe that a Power greater than myself could restore me to sanity.*

I guess I could compare insanity to my natural fallen state. Sanity then is the atonement taking effect in my life one defect at a time. As the atonement takes away each defect a step and a day at a time, I am restored to sanity.

Who am I to think that my defects are beyond the saving grace of Christ who has promised that He has the power to redeem everyone—one person at a time, one defect at a time? Certainly I have known this for many years and yet I continued to believe that I was meant to have the eating defect so I wallowed in it. Why would I think that? I don't really know except that perhaps I had not truly acknowledged the love of Christ for me. The past couple years I have taken time to notice and give thanks for His many tender mercies to me, just keeping from gaining weight is a tremendous blessing and evidence of His power reaching out to save me from food hell. It is this power that has kept me from using food to cope with the stresses in my life. Though troubled on every side I am not distressed—perplexed at times but not in despair as Paul [New Testament apostle] said.

# After all I can do

Nov 14, 2007

The words that I have underlined in the bible dictionary definition of grace are: help, strength, assistance, enabling power, and His grace cannot suffice without total effort on my part.

I guess what I may find confusing in this definition is what exactly is total effort on my part. How much is total effort and how is that measured? How will I know when I have given my total effort? How will I know when I have done all I can do?

I know that I need His help and strength and enabling power and assistance and I know that it is available to me. I just don't know when I've done my part and when He takes over.

I also know that my body is sacred and certainly caring for it fits the criteria for a 'good work'. I know that my past behavior has demonstrated that I don't have the power to carry on this good work of caring for my body for any great length of time before I weary in well-doing and resort to the comfort of eating. I just don't know when I can say that I have given my total effort in maintaining my health. Does it mean that I regularly engage in exercise along with three moderate meals a day? Does it mean that I don't eat any sugar or refined carbs of any sort? Does it mean that I don't eat after 6 pm or that I eat only in response to hunger? I guess I'm having trouble defining what my effort should be and what exactly abstinence means to me.

My faith in Christ has always provided me with peace and security. It is my ultimate hope that all will be well in my life but when I feel my peace and security threatened with lack of self-confidence in making money decisions, doubts creep in, my confidence wanes, and my mouth opens wide to accept whatever is available to put into it.

November, 2007

As far as my addiction to food goes, I have yet to have long term abstinence. I have experienced months at a time but somehow transition times seem to call me back to the familiarity of food. I would like to have turning to God whenever these uncertain times come as my automatic response rather than turning to food. I would like the assurance and testimony of knowing that I will not succumb to the addiction no matter what may be happening in my life. Is that too much to want?

It is still the desire and question that I have sitting there on my abdominal shelf with all the other mysteries I have waiting to be answered someday.

# What would Jesus eat?

Has anyone else noticed that food seems to be the center of almost everything we do in this food prosperous society? Food is ubiquitous. If you want a crowd to show up, bring food and make it free and fattening and fast.

November, 2007

*Now let's take the guy full of faith, but still reeking of alcohol* (or the woman who is full of faith but more full of food on a chronic basis). For some reason this line stood out to me as I paraphrased it and was reminded of my many eating orgies associated with church functions. In fact, how many have I been to that food was my only motivation for going and how many firesides or baptisms or leadership meetings did I attend only to find with great disappointment that there was NO FOOD (it's enough to make a person apostatize)? Sad isn't it, that so much emphasis has been placed on the pleasure of food rather than the joy of the Spirit. Why do people come for the food but not for the Spirit? What is even more sad is that the 'food' served at these various functions is so far removed from actual food that it kills more than it nourishes and yet we have the audacity to ask God to bless it to nourish and strengthen our bodies. Why do we do that? It's about as insane as addiction. I wonder what God thinks of it. I wonder if He's up there shaking His head and thinking 'there's no way I can bless that to nourish and strengthen your bodies or I would cease to be God.'

I have often paraphrased the scripture, 'Where two or three are gathered in His name, there is food in the midst of them,' and we are so focused on the food and stuffing ourselves that we fail to notice that He is there. He is there and no one noticed because the donuts or rice crispy squares or brownies were a bigger hit.

The word 'fight' is how I have chronically felt about my battle with food. There have been times that I honestly looked forward to having a famine in the land so that food would not be around to torment me and I would finally be rid of it and the thighs that go with it. When I was a missionary in refugee camps in Thailand I remember talking to Cambodian refugees about the western obsession with dieting. They were so shocked that people would have to intentionally not eat to avoid getting fat. The idea that food abundance would be a problem seemed totally foreign to them and I guess it was because in their culture it didn't hold that power. This was the first time I realized that, for much of the world's population, food is scarce and hard to get and the fight is to get enough for survival. Yet in prosperous nations there is abundance and the fight is to avoid excess. There's something wrong with this picture for sure.

There is still something wrong with that picture. In North America obesity continues to be a huge health problem, while outside North America millions are starving to death. I suppose one could say that obese people are also starving in their own way, suffering from lack of nutritious food while stuffing themselves with fake food.

# Eating Utensils

In the next entry I list and ruminate on the tools of recovery.

November, 2007

Abstinence:

I know that when I indulge in excess food, especially junk food, I become irritable, negative, fearful, down, and pessimistic—all those things associated with lack of faith and an absence of the Spirit. I'm not sure why this is. I just know that it is. I've experienced enough excess then abstinence from sugar to know the effect it has on me, yet sometimes I still find myself wallowing in the mire of sugar. When I'm away from the addiction I feel powerful, strong, confident, hopeful, and able to do all things, then something happens that flips me back head first into a bag of chips or some sort of junk. There I am again, self-loathing and despondent. The more I am abstinent, the more I want to be so my willingness is definitely increased.

Literature:

Reading motivating literature is definitely a powerful tool for me and can change my body chemistry and motives in a flash. I have for many years known the power in the *Book of Mormon* to alter my moods, motives, and actions. I am exercising faith now that it will help to remove the desire to eat in a self-destructive way. I have recently had an epiphany about the *New Testament* story of the woman who had the issue with blood and had been to many specialists to heal her then touched the hem of Christ's garment and was healed. I am the woman with an issue with food and I have tried many worldly experts' solutions to no avail. Like the woman in the *New Testament*, I feel that if I can just get close enough to Christ I will be healed, as she was. It is the knowledge of and repetition of such literature that gradually increases my belief that God can and will remove the self-destructive habits I have.

Writing:

I have had experiences where I have been able to diffuse many a stressful situation through writing. I have also frequently written long enough that the frustrations, fears, and disappointments have turned into prayers and I have felt the tension give way to comfort and solace. Writing is also one place where I can be brutally honest without offending anyone or getting into trouble for speaking my mind. It's one of those places where thoughts and feelings are unleashed without any fear of reprisal or regret for venting.

Prayer and meditation:

The only way to know God is to be in touch with Him on a continual basis. Some of my most profound and meaningful epiphanies have come to me when I have been praying vocally while walking through the woods, or meditating and pondering on some scripture or event, or playing my piano and singing. The more prayerful I am, the more these epiphany moments occur, giving me the warm assurance that God really does like me. I have grown used to experiencing these regularly and when a few days go by that I don't feel a connection with God then I am frightened and insecure (these usually happen when I have descended once again into food hell). One day after a few days of food hell and distancing from God, I once again felt that unmistakable peace that only God gives. I was so relieved and said to God, 'I'm so glad you're back'. The immediate Heavenly response was, 'No, I'm glad YOU'RE back. I wasn't the one who went away, it was you'. Then I know that I am once again with God, not the world.

As for me and my house, we will serve food.

November, 2007

Over the years, as I have observed the effects of various foods on my spiritual and physical health, I have realized that there is tremendous power for good or evil in food and fake food. The food that comes of the earth as God intended it to come is both physically and spiritually nourishing, while the food that comes from men's processing and pulverizing and enriching is not. These 'food' items, aptly termed 'junk' food, not only don't nourish, but also sap the body and spirit of its health and ability to be one with God.

What I am puzzled about though is why, generally speaking, is our social focus in the church so much to do with dead food? Think of those potluck salads, casseroles etc. that contain no visible actual food items. Am I getting a bit too cynical or do we worship food more than we do God? Or is it just me that is worshipping food rather than God, or am I just getting off on another compulsive obsessive tangent?

If food has such power to nourish or to kill, then it does not surprise me that God would be interested in what I eat. Naturally He would counsel and empower me in my eating behaviors. Physical nourishment is at the core of human survival, and God is all about keeping people alive eternally, both body and spirit together as the soul of man. In short, I have found that food has the power to connect or disconnect me from God.

If God cares about what I eat, He obviously cares about what I think and do and say and sing and wear. I trust in Him to have all things work together for my good as I accept whatever is His will and allow Him to fight my battles including the battle of the bulge.

# Buns of buns

<u>December, 2007</u>

I've had a pattern for years of eating excessively when things don't go as I want them to go. Even when things go how I want them to go, I have been known to eat to excess. With Christmas coming on, I am reminded of my failure with marriage. It seems that Christmas is the one time more than any other that I miss being married and I miss the log home where I raised my children and how beautiful it was with my Christmas decorations in it. I would have to say then that at this time of year I am not content with the way things are, even though I know that the discontent will pass. There is something about Christmas that makes most people want a cozy loving family sitting around the fireplace (and I did have one in my home as a married person).

So it shouldn't be a surprise that I am thinking about those cinnamon rolls that the neighbor brought over yesterday and I'm almost convinced that eating them all will give me the sense that I am back in my log home, and it is decorated beautifully, and all is well with the world for the time.

A rational person will know that those cinnamon rolls have nothing to do with my marital status or my contentment or the way my house is decorated. They aren't love or peace or joy or family and I'm pretty sure they weren't part of the original Christmas with Mary and Joseph and Jesus, so I am giving them much more power than they deserve?

December, 2007

I want God to change my heart so I know that I will never again engage in compulsive overeating and that I will eat rationally and in a manner to promote optimum health for my body and spirit. I want Him to take away my obsession with myself and my cellulite and my 'do I look fat in this' complex. Deliverance from an obsession with self would be a blessing.

# Fit for the Kingdom?

December, 2007

The Word of Wisdom is full of things to avoid (alcohol, tobacco, excess meat, hot drinks, interpreted as tea and coffee) and I easily avoid all these things. From my birth my parents gave me a perfect model for avoiding such harmful substances. These substances are not now, nor have they ever been, a temptation to me. However avoiding excess food, which is also part of this revelation, has been a struggle for me. I know that if I start eating refined carbs and any kind of processed foods I will overindulge. I can overindulge on nutritious food too, but not so much so as with refined foods. I believe that the Word of Wisdom also teaches this with its admonition to eat whole foods, fruit, and plants.

The cognitive dissonance comes when all the treats and junk are accepted in our religion and yet are being shown to be equally as harmful as the other forbidden substances (think obesity being the new tobacco).

I'm getting more and more confused about this and know that if the ward Christmas party did not include a food spread of fattening goodies, there are those who would be so offended that they would never show up to church again. What does all that rich food have to do with the birth of Christ? When I admit that I don't do any Christmas baking some people are so appalled that you'd think I crucified Christ because I'm not stocking my house with shortbread and fudge and fruit cake to celebrate His birth. Alas, I am suffering from acute cognitive dissonance wanting to indulge in the fat of Christmas yet knowing those time tested traditions will only remove me from the very Person whose birth is being celebrated and who alone can deliver me from the madness of food.

# The many chins of Eve

<u>December, 2007</u>

I have most definitely fallen prey to (and continue to be enticed by) every wind of doctrine in the dieting world. You'd think that by now I would have learned that every new miracle diet is just another spin off of the old diets and yet they all sound so inviting. I have realized that I am just as addicted to dieting as I am to food, and of course this time of year gets me in an absolute frenzy of cognitive dissonance where food and dieting is concerned. The thrill of mentally romancing another crash diet is just as exciting as the thrill of romancing another binge (of course last night's ward Christmas dinner was the binge to end all binges). While I was falling prey to the notion that this binge really would end all binges, I am simultaneously planning the diet to end all diets. Is this madness or what? Just who ARE these disparate people living in my body? It's getting awfully crowded in my head and body and pants. But of course, the cabbage soup diet could end all that, couldn't it? Why don't I do something different this year and start the diet before Christmas rather than after the New Year? That way I can drop a few pounds fast before the biggest binge day of the year, binge one day, then be back in fine form to start the New Year. Ah, my carnal nature. It's still there and I still need the atonement and repentance and meetings and abstinence and food.

Sometime during the Christmas season I lost contact with my sponsor. She never responded to my last exercise submission and I assumed she was done with me. Of course I did not pursue the sponsoring relationship further, being concerned that she no longer may have had time for me.

I managed to maintain reasonable abstinence through to the end of the year, largely because I had a special education colloquium to attend in California during the final week of the year and I did not want to feel fat for it. I held it together until the last day when I ordered an abundance of food via room service to celebrate alone on New Year's Eve.

I had injured my ankle while running in California and lay in my hotel room with my foot up, chewing the fat. When the waiter took my phone order, he asked how many sets of utensils and plates I needed. There was an awkward silence when I said only one. The message was clear: I was eating way too much food for just one person. I was officially in binge mode to end the year, alone in a hotel room in Anaheim, California. Alas, I was still me, damn it! And I was still writing wonderful goals for change, all the while stuffing myself with an amount of food that could clearly have fed many more than me. Need I say more? My journal entry that night is just as disorganized as was my binging.

> December 31, 2007 Anaheim, California 5:00 a.m.
>
> What and who do I want to be?
>
> It's about the spirit growing and the body shrinking (literally) or about having more of God and less of

me. I give myself to God and He gives me back better, more powerful, more intelligent, more beautiful, more joyful, more loving, more serene, more lovable, more enjoyable, more holy, more like Him because I have willingly given over myself to Him. My body becomes the way He created it—not polluted and distorted through the excesses of the world.

He has rescued me and continues to rescue me daily from my own follies and foibles and food fits and ignorance.

## Eat, drink, and be miserable.

Back home in Creston, I started another teaching contract with the college. The darkness of winter was all around, and I could not walk it off with my injured ankle. Without my walk therapy the descent into food hell was at record speed, even for me. Clinging to prayer, I desperately pleaded for it to be otherwise. But I knew my heart was really not in the lip service I gave to God. Huckleberry Finn comes to mind. All the while praying, I was planning the next food I would eat as soon as I got off my knees. I knew I couldn't pray a lie, but still desperately tried.

<u>January 10, 2008 6:15 a.m.</u>

I've been awake reading my *Book of Mormon* since 5:00 a.m. searching for that peace that I have been missing the past few weeks as I have once again descended into sugar/food hell. O Lord, be merciful unto such a sinner as myself. After reading Alma's writings to his sons, I am reminded that I have been allowing pride to surface again—pride and bitterness. I desperately need God in my life and have felt disconnected again. All the old feelings of fear, anxiety, loneliness, and insecurity have come rushing in on me and with them a panic to eat in an attempt to assuage the negative feelings. It is not coincidental that these feelings have come during a time that I have not been able to get out and walk on a regular basis. Physical exercise is essential to mental and spiritual health. I haven't been sleeping as well either so as soon as I get fatigued I feel crappy and reach for junk food. Does that make any sense?

It's like I get going on this downward spiral of insecurities, doubts, fears, and such, with poor sleep, little exercise, and slothfulness again with spiritual habits as well.

Then last night I went off to my food addiction meeting in the hopes that this would inject new hope into my flagging soul, but there were only two of us who showed up. Neither of us had a chapel key with us so we chatted briefly then went home. I baked some cookie dough (stuff I had from a Christmas fundraising project), and ate about a dozen cookies while watching the news. Of course that made me feel worse, going to bed stuffed with cookies. How pathetic am I?

# Awake my soul; no longer droop in sugar

Jan 18, 2008

My emotions continue to be from one extreme to the other. It is only by the grace of God that I am able to function daily in my job and school and other demands of life. Thankfully to God my ankle has stood up to a daily walk and that has helped me tremendously in coping with whatever is going on in my head and heart and everywhere else. I must be honest and say that the excess sugar is NOT helping. On Monday we went to the DQ. There was a special on dilly bars—buy one box and get a second free. So what does any budget-conscious food-storing Mormon do? Buy the deal, and I did eat. So I've been eating several dilly bars every day and hating myself in every bite.

I've bounced from feelings of total despair, insecurity, and hopelessness to lesser versions of the same. I've probably got some menopause induced emotions going on too, but certainly these are exacerbated by my abysmal eating habits.

Help me Lord for I am definitely in the gall of bitterness and dwelling on all that I have done wrong in life, all that I feel is unfair in life, and imagining more despair and grief. It's basically been like Nephi's (*Book of Mormon* prophet) "O wretched man that I am" week. This morning I was awake at 4:00 a.m. feeling frightened, alone, remorseful, and abandoned by God, so I did the only thing I know of that really helps in situations like this—I opened my *Book of Mormon* and began to read. This time I was in Alma 41 verse 7, "delivered from that endless night of darkness." As the verses carry on, Alma discusses the power of choice and desire to take us where we want to be, happy or miserable. Perhaps I have not made it clear to myself that I do want happiness and not misery. Sugar never was happiness, never has been, and never will be. Junk food never was happiness, never has been, and never will be.

I suppose I'm also feeling some sadness that Alicia is growing up and I no longer have a child who wants to be with me. Perhaps I'm starting to realize that I am alone and this aloneness is compounded when I remove myself from God through my own actions and choices and vain imaginations of bitterness.

I have also not been sleeping as well as I need and that compounds all the other problems. Of course the poor sleeping is also related to the excess sugar and snacking in the evening. It's a vicious cycle of self-pity and destruction and today I hope to get off it by first getting off the sugar.

February 3, 2008

Several weeks have gone by again. More snow falls. Last weekend I took Alicia to Calgary to try out for a volleyball team so we spent Friday and Saturday nights there. She played volleyball most of Saturday and Sunday morning. I sat and read assignments for my two courses. We went to Costco and got a huge supply of food essentials and some non-essentials. I ate a lot of junk food and felt like crap most of the weekend. We drove home in a snowstorm.

Somewhere between morning and night the mood shifted once again and I was off sugar for a brief time.

February 2008

I have once again got off sugar and refined carbs. My mood has been so up and down throughout January and a large part of that is because of what I have been eating. I know that sugar affects my emotions and motivation. When I get stuck in sugar hell, I feel negative, despairing, lonely, anxious and fearful about life. When I get off the sugar and junk I notice an immediate elevation in my mood and a far greater sense of hope and confidence for the future.

I am so happy to be off sugar again this past week and hope that I can remember the awfulness of being on it to keep me from indulging and descending down again into sugar hell. It seems that when I start worrying about my children and dwelling on my past mistakes that I start wallowing in self-pity then I don't like myself so I get into junk again with that 'who cares' attitude. On the other hand, when I remember all that God has blessed me with and how He has carried me through the troubles in my life, I feel optimistic about the future, and the loneliness and fear leave me.

### February 17, 2008

I have been sick this weekend with a sore throat and cough. I really got in a self-pity mode today at church, feeling despairing and the usual negativism. I'll feel better when this cold is gone and I get outside and start walking again. My confidence is suffering and I want to curl up somewhere and hide or eat myself into a coma.

It seemed that I stressed myself needlessly with taking on extra school and projects. I am not sure why I did that. Having too much on my metaphorical life plate always seemed to coincide with having too much on my food plate. Living life in a frenzy taking big gulps translated into eating food in a frenzy of big gulps. The bigger my plate, the bigger my butt.

### March 9, 2008

I will be finished my two courses next Friday and what a relief that will be. I have felt very stressed with the workload and have been eating to excess. That's an indication that I am feeling overwhelmed and my clothes are getting tight and it's time to get a handle on things again.

Well, let's see what else I can talk about here. Along with my excess disordered eating, I have become more negative and critical and fearful of finances and future etc.

All areas of my life seemed to fall apart when eating fell apart. My life really was unmanageable.

March 14, 2008

What a relief it is to have my two courses done and a few weeks off from schooling. All my children are home this weekend. Right now they're out. It's time to reflect and remind myself of the joys of spirituality over carnality. Joan has been cleaning my house for me and organizing closets and such. I am in a very slovenly state and plan to spend tomorrow dunging out, taking garbage to the dump, and cleaning my filthy car. I'm ashamed at how messy things are right now and it all coincides with my out-of-control eating. It's ridiculous how disordered and insane I get with eating—totally ridiculous.

Here comes another dieting frenzy to go with the life frenzy. I was eternally seeking that quick fix to an eternal problem. My cognitive dissonance is screaming.

March 23, 2008

This past week I have been doing the cabbage soup diet. Today is the last day and I must say that I feel better than I did last week. I want to conquer my food addiction. I know that I am powerless over it and can overcome it only through the mercy and grace of Christ. I love my body and want to take care of it. Sugar is a very destructive substance to me and I have known this for many years and yet I continue to falter when I let my guard down and begin to think that it really isn't that bad for me. I want to be fit and beautiful without excess flab. I know that it is only through Christ's grace that I will actually achieve the power to conquer my carnal excesses.

# To every season there is a diet

There is nothing like the arrival of spring after a long dark Canadian winter to lift flagging spirits and bring a renewal of hope for the chronic dieter. Something in the air just reeks of hope and lightens the misery of food darkness.

<u>April 30, 2008</u>

I am feeling good tonight after having gone to the food addiction meeting. I am feeling a renewal of hope and commitment to the program and genuinely wanting to once again work through the steps after having spent some time eating indiscriminately and excessively. I had several wonderful walks today though it continues to be quite cold and not feeling very spring like yet.

It's clear that I was trying desperately to replace one compulsion with another. Compulsive exercise certainly was better than compulsive eating. With the longer days I could hide out outside away from the awfulness of the kitchen.

<u>May 3, 2008</u>

Yesterday I walked out to mom's after work (about four miles) and visited for a while then walked back. It was a good workout. Today I walked to work, walked on my lunch break, walked home, then walked for an hour with my neighbor. I'm back to being motivated to get the weight off again. I've probably gained ten pounds again this winter. Ugh. I wonder how long it's going to take for me to really change and not relapse back to binge eating. Today I feel good having had such good walks as well as a physically active work day. I started another marker for abstinence on May 1st and I am grateful to God for His sustenance thus far.

That abstinence was short lived, the agony of relapse written once again on paper and on my thighs for all to see.

May 28, 2008

I just got back from a church women's meeting on preparedness. I feel sad thinking of the physical security I felt in my home in Lister and the days of gardening and root cellars. I feel disorganized, unprepared, alone, and fat. I've been eating excessively for over a week now. I'm scared of my carnal urge to eat to excess. I'm afraid of getting fat, depressed, lethargic, and undesirable.

I'm 52 years old and here I am still struggling with the same carnal issues I had 35 years ago. It's getting exhausting dealing with the same food issues over and over and over again. I could sit and eat 'til I'm sick. Why, why, why?

Do I hate myself? Do I want to destroy myself? I'm not stupid, so why can't I overcome this weakness, Lord? I want to be lean and healthy. I want to have a healthy relationship with food. I'm scared of food. Why am I scared of food? It's just food. What's wrong with me Lord? I don't seem to be able to beat this.

With the relapse came the inevitable consequence—more migraine misery.

June 2, 2008

Oh Lord, thank Thee for this day of migraine misery, nausea, and vomiting to remind me why I don't want junk food and excess in my life.

Enter the raw food diet, raw and short lived. I'm not even sure why I started this one except that one of my students was doing it and testifying to its marvelous weight loss results.

June 10, 2008

I'm grateful to still be eating raw and feeling very good about it.

The size of my body seemed to influence so many other things in my life—where I went, what I did, how I served, how I worshipped, who I liked and disliked.

June 11, 2008

I had a food addiction meeting tonight. We're starting to use the church approved addiction program. Our bishop was at the chapel for a meeting and came in to say hi then asked me to give a talk in church next month. I told him that I have a suit I want to get into before I speak again. He laughed and said that I have 1½ months to get into it.

Mormon bishops' counsel is something to be revered and respected. The suit never fit that summer, but I accepted the assignment from my bishop anyway. I also took the opportunity to ask the bishop if he noticed I am overweight just so

I could say that I had confessed to my bishop. He laughed in response and I knew what that meant. 'Nuff said!

## Just say no already!

In June 2008 I went with my daughter on a volleyball trip to Reno. The trip was more than I could afford, but saying no to my children never seemed to be an easy thing for me. I was about as good at saying no to them as I was at saying no to food. Wonder what the connection is there!?

July 2, 2008

> Rather disappointing week and expensive too. I wish I was home. No volleyball today. We all went to Lake Tahoe for awhile. I felt fat and sloppy but put on my bathing suit and walked in the water for awhile. It's been very difficult having any control over events here, i.e. when to eat and stuff. I can't wait to get home.

Later that summer, my daughter went off to train with the BC volleyball team and I had some time alone. Foremost in my thoughts was how much weight I might lose while she was gone.

July 13, 2008

> I am all alone for the next two weeks and am hoping to lose ten pounds eating grass, fruit, and nuts.

<u>July 20, 2008</u>

I've been doing well with my food habits this past week. It's much easier to manage food intake being by myself.

The summer past and with it the food plan and weight loss hopes. My house was filled with incoming and outgoing family and guests and food. What's a compulsive over-eater to do? Eat until the house was quiet again.

<u>August 24, 2008</u>

The house is quiet again. Yesterday Alicia and I shovelled out the house. I don't know why I let the house get so messy. My slob demon is as hard to fight as my food demon.

<u>September 14, 2008</u>

This past week I've been pondering over why I am so slovenly and why it was so hard for me to keep an orderly home.

I want to have a house of order as much as I want to overcome my sugar addiction.

Neither one has been conquered but daily reprieve is all I can hope for now. I could just hire a housekeeper and solve one problem, but hiring a 24/7 person to manage my food intake would be way beyond my budget, besides being an impossible task.

# Diet hard or go home!

The fall has always seemed more to me like the New Year than January. It's when everything seems to start up again—school, work, and diets to get ready for Christmas. 2008 was the start of yoga for me. Actually it was yoga revisited. I did some yoga back in my twenties, about 28 days to be exact, and then I stretched myself right on out of there and into another fad.

September 16, 2008

I've bought a yoga book and have started doing some yoga poses for flexibility. I used to do yoga years ago in my twenties. Just think how good I could be if I continued these past thirty years. Ah well, I have started again.

I'm grateful for a week of abstinence from sugar and compulsive eating. Life is much more peaceful this way.

September 17, 2008

I'm awake and feeling light and happy for not eating last night. The young women at church had snacks for their activity and I abstained from all of them. What a blessing it is to awaken and know that I did not pollute my body yesterday. I have the feeling of hope and peace that come from abstinence from sugar and all refined food products. I look forward to the day with eager anticipation of what it will bring.

October 9, 2008

Today is my 53rd birthday and I'm reflecting on what I still look forward to doing with my life. I still have my food issues but have not had refined sugar for a month now. I have baked with Splenda and pigged out on dried prunes so still have food issues. I am hoping as I explore my past doing research for a dissertation I may resolve some of those issues and lay them to rest and move on.

Not much changed in me as I continued to go round and round the misery go round of food addiction. I'm getting nauseated just reading about it but then again, not so nauseated that I can't eat.

October 10, 2008

I am struggling to get food obsession out of my life. My carnal nature is rearing its ugly head once again. Maybe if I bike long enough I'll at least be distracted for the moment. Just for today I'll eat what I need to glorify rather than gorge my body.

9:30 p.m. I got the ingredients for my Thanksgiving dessert then watched a dumb movie. It was really stupid actually. I ate too much. I am struggling big time with food.

October 12, 2008

Two scriptures testify and promise, "Because thou hast seen thy weakness, thou shalt be made strong" Ether

12: 57 in the *Book of Mormon* and section 135 verse 5 in the *Doctrine and Covenants*.

Lord, I see my weakness for excess food. I see my gluttony and my weakness for using food for love, hate, and boredom. Please make me strong so that food becomes only nourishment as my body needs it, that my body will be as Thou hast meant for it to be.

I am amazed at the level of fitness I maintained and yet still hung onto my fat. Isn't there something wrong with this picture? In the words of Erma Bombeck, you'd think I should be hanging from a charm bracelet by now!

October 13, 2008

I am totally exhausted from our extreme hike today— 10.4 kilometres to the Thompson Mountain lookout and then another 10.4 kilometres back down. It was a church ward fitness challenge. It took about six hours to go up and back down. I've been totally exhausted since and now in pain.
Besides that I've got terrible gas from the maltelol sweetened chocolates Alicia gave me and the dried prunes I binged on. I feel totally drained.

October 14, 2008

Here's another day to repent of my carnal self. Just for today I will use food for its purpose: to glorify rather than gorge my body.

# In my mind's thigh

You gotta hand it to me. I was really good at writing goals. I had it down to a fine science and left no fat cell unturned. I rocked at writing goals and daily plans and grandiose visualizations.

October 15, 2008

I'm thinking of an LDS apostle's conference talk on creating the day spiritually before it happens. So this is how I would create my day spiritually.

1. start with reading the *Book of Mormon* (done)
2. have a good walk
3. eat eggs and fruit shake for breakfast.
4. go to work, treat all people with respect, be authentic in all communication and generous with praise, no sarcasm
5. lunch: eat bean casserole with cheese on top, go for a walk to the health store and buy evening primrose oil to ease my hormone transitions
6. off work at 5 p.m. then go for a brisk walk, and have turkey soup supper
7. take Alicia to volleyball then go to my food addiction meeting

Eat only at specified meals sitting down and enjoying. Eat nothing after 6 p.m. Enjoy going to bed with an empty stomach.

10:00 p.m. How it actually went:

I was abstinent today from compulsive eating and for that I thank God. I believe I was authentic and genuine in communication and treated others respectfully. I went to a meeting tonight with just one other person there but feel inspired. I am ready for bed now with my hot water bottle.

October 18, 2008

Today I want to ponder peaceful thoughts and live just for today. I want to abstain from compulsive overeating. Yesterday at work I read a handout on bladder problems. Sugar is listed as an irritant to the urinary bladder, so is caffeine. There's another reason to abstain. So for those suffering with urinary tract infections or overactive bladder, it is recommended they cut out sugar and caffeine (chocolate, pop, coffee etc.). I am thankful for these messages from God all around me.

October 21, 2008 3:30 a.m.

I've been awake for an hour now with a rumbling belly from eating in the evening and maybe too many beans. I know that eating and drinking in the evening is disruptive to my sleep so exactly WHY do I continue to do it? I have a scripture playing in my head, "Thy neck is an iron sinew". How many times does it take to get it?

October 25, 2008

I continue to eat nutritiously. The more I read the more convinced I am not to eat sugar.

<u>November 5, 2008</u>

I am regretting some things I said from yesterday so I'll get that all off my thighs before getting out in the world today.

If only life would not get in the way of my goals and plans and programs and lists and visualizations, I could be the center of the universe and all would be well. If life were like that I wouldn't have ever needed a diet in the first place.

# The fatter I get, the thinner I was

Not much to say but watch as I continued to expand once again, mad at every pound added yet still trying to cling to the size I was. The fatter I got, the thinner I was.

November 9, 2008

Friday I insisted on wearing my old size ten jeans (have nothing else), which are too small. After suffering a few hours I went over to Winners between volleyball games and bought a new pair (size twelve). I kept remembering a piece of fashion advice I read somewhere, "No matter what size you are, you look better in clothes that fit."

I felt much better with my new jeans but annoyed with myself for expanding.

November 10, 2008

Alicia asked me why women gain so much weight after getting married noting specific women who had gained after marriage, yet they were both so trim when they married. I'm not sure why getting fat seems to go along with having and raising a family. Part of it is being around food so much and preparing food it seems, constantly for children. Obviously eating too many refined and packaged foods is also a big problem. Weight has always been an issue for me and I can empathize with those women who have gained weight.

I spent great blocks of time trying to analyze my habits and patterns of behaviors trying to identify just when my brain switch went from super health nut to totally debauched binging freak. For this binge the catalyst was a flood in my kitchen. It was another glitch in my perfectly laid out plans.

December 6, 2008

Anatomy of a binge:

Yesterday while the workers tore up my flood-damaged flooring I spent the time holed up in my computer room researching for my dissertation. When I realized I was hungry after noon I couldn't get to my kitchen and the fridge was blocked off and the workers were busy. Prior to this, my neighbor had delivered cinnamon buns to us for Christmas. All I had (conveniently) were those cinnamon buns so in my hunger I ate five of them. Ugh! Later I went out for a walk to try to mitigate some of the harmful effects. Later, after picking up Alicia and her friend, we picked up convenience food at the grocery store—fried chicken and potato wedges and some salad— and ate too much. I feel like crap this morning.

# The morning after diet

My life was either feast or fast. I'm not sure why. There's only a one letter difference between those two words, and yet what a vast chasm that meant between the fat feasting me and the fit fasting me. For me, the E in feast stands for EAT and that's what I did. I changed so fast from one to the other that even I wasn't sure who, the eater or the faster, was there inside of me on any given day.

<u>December 7, 2008 7:30 a.m.</u>

I'm grateful for my fasting. I can wake up without that icky feeling of having pigged out last night. The sugar demon reared its ugly head again propelled by the cinnamon bun binge. I hope this fast will subdue the demon once again.

<u>December 9, 2008</u>

I awakened early, probably because my digestive system hasn't been resting. My neck is an iron sinew and I wonder, will I ever learn? Will I ever internalize what I know and act on it (speaking of eating, I mean)?

Not only was my neck an iron sinew, but my thighs as well. The power of eating was much more powerful than me and I continued to seek a Power greater than myself to conquer it.

Dear God,

I'm sorry I've been such a carnal creature and have once again descended into sugar hell. I want to be free from sugar addiction. I want to take care of my body. I love my body. It does marvellous things for me. I'm sorry for the insults I have placed on my temple, the desecration of excess food piled up after overworking my liver and pancreas and stomach and bowels. Why do I do this self-abuse and torture?

December 11, 2008

I went to the Spokane temple today. After the temple we stopped briefly at Costco and I got some cord pants. Now I've got some pants that fit my expanded size. How do I let myself gain weight over and over again? Yesterday I got off sugar again and already feel much better. One day at a time.

As another year came to a close I totally succumbed to the excesses of the season.

December 27, 2008

We have lots of snow. I'm overfed, over dosed on sugar, and undernourished. Ugh! I can't believe how far I've fallen into food hell again. I wonder how I get myself into such terrible holes again. I feel exhausted though today I did get out for a couple walks in the snow.

I worked the 25th and 26th and was surrounded by junk food at work. I'm definitely removed from my spiritual source and the grace of God.

Don't you just love the end of a year when hope springs eternal that something magic will happen on New Year's Eve, that some magical angel will touch your brain and body and turn you into the person of your dreams in the twinkling of a fat cell? What would I do without my yearly resolution rituals that promise to make me free from my fat self?

December 31, 2008

I went grocery shopping to stock up on veggies and nutritious food. It's time to cast off the junk of the season.

So here's the year in review: 2008

Physically: My weight has increased somewhat and I am wearing size twelve pants instead of size ten. I don't know my actual weight because I'm afraid to stand on the scale. I continued to walk regularly but I know I have descended into food hell many times this past year and as a result have gradually expanded in width.

So what do I hope for in 2009? I hope that when 2009 comes to its close I will be a comfortable size eight. To accomplish my goals I will once again give up sugar and junk food, pay strict attention to what I eat, as well as give strict attention to the twelve-step program and tools while continuing to attend meetings. Progress seems to be a circular rather than linear process.

# Faceweight.com

Every New Year's Eve seemed to turn into the binge to end all binges and this one was no different. The only thing that stopped my binging was falling asleep. Every New Year's Day promised to be the purge to end all purges.

January 1, 2009

I ate junk and junk and more junk last night. I am so ready to move on, flush out the crap, and move forward to once again focus on health and spirituality. So today I'm having a fruit day to rest my poor body.

Two days into the New Year and I was off to watch my superstar son play in a university volleyball tournament. Two days into my new diet plan I was eating again without restraint.

January 3, 2009

After the volleyball game we were invited to a local home, one of the player's families, for a party. There was lots of food and I did eat. Not even sure why, but it was delicious.

January 4, 2009

I had an epiphany for a website yesterday—Faceweight.com. As I sat on the toilet contemplating my weight woes I thought maybe I should go on Facebook and declare my weight openly. Then it hit me that this might be a great tool for others wanting to discuss weight issues and get support while sharing their pictures as they struggle and lose weight. Faceweight seemed a good name.

Armed with my indestructible optimism and a new workout plan, I persevered onward and downward with the numbers on the scale. My oldest daughter introduced me to the Slim in Six workout DVDs and I started these with great anticipation of the lean me that would emerge in this, the year I would finally arrive.

<u>January 5, 2009</u>

I thought of a quotation that has something to do with jealousy or admiration, whichever way you look at it. I see others having what I don't but they're doing what I'm not. This could apply to women with great bodies, great minds, education, spirituality etc.
Rather than envy those people, see what they're doing and do it too.
I want 2009 to be the year that I shake off the chains of food hell, build muscle, and love my body.

<u>January 8, 2009</u>

Thank Thee for where I am today, for another day of deliverance from overeating and another day of abstinence from sugar and junk food. Thank Thee for health and for my heritage of healthy habits.
Joan is teaching me about fitness tapes. I'm doing one to trim down along with my walking.

# Ruthless bludgeoning

With relapse comes a significant amount of self-bludgeoning over the stupidity of being on the misery go around of dieting and binging. Writing out the misery kept me from eating into the dark hole of wherever I was inclined to go with my food-fuelled self-hatred.

January 9, 2009

This past week I've been very mad at myself for once again food binging and gaining weight. I'm not going to step on the scale because I know it will depress me but I've probably put on twenty pounds this past year. Once again I'm wondering what I was thinking. It's probably the worst binging I've done in years. The old food demons returned and I don't know why. Anyway, Oprah also has gained again, forty pounds she says and now she's also mad too. I wonder how she can have so much trouble when she has so much money and resources supplying her with top world experts in diet, exercise, and obesity. This morning I was once again bemoaning this and saying she has all those experts helping her and she can't do it. What have I got in comparison? Immediately the epiphany hit and the Spirit said, "You've got God." What more do I need and what would I rather have, the experts of the world or God?

This morning I was reading an LDS apostle's conference talk on angels. He was discussing how each of us goes through periods of despair and darkness but God has angels (sometimes ordinary people) to get us through the dark spells. I know that even during these dark winter months there is sure to be spring and longer brighter days coming soon. I have hope that even though I have once again plunged into the dark abyss of food excess and fat, I will come out of this abyss into the leaner me by spring. The lean me is the real me—the me that God created. The fat me is the distortions I have created by distancing myself from the Creator.

By the look of my journaling, I got through January on a prayer and a workout. Actually, it was more like several prayers and several workouts.

January 12, 2009

I've had a good week of deliverance from overeating and have done the first six days of the Slim in Six video workouts.

January 13, 2009

I am grateful for a week of deliverance from overeating. I am reading in scripture this morning about singing a new song. Here is my new diet song:
"Oh Lord, according to my faith in Thee wilt Thou deliver me from this pride in my heart before it destroys my soul and give me strength to burst these food bands with which I am bound?" Of course I

am paraphrasing Nephi and Jacob (*Book of Mormon* prophets), but it seems to have worked for them, so it should work for me.

# Write it off

For some reason 2009 was a losing year for me, losing being a good thing in this case. My journal entries are filled with the praise of freedom from feasting to excess.

<u>January 14, 2009</u>

I feel like I've spent most of my life doing what other people want. Now that I'm very close to being on my own with my children adults I want to honor what I genuinely want to do and to be.
I'm angry after browsing a book claiming to reveal part of my family history so I'm going to write instead of eat.

<u>January 19, 2009 7:00 a.m.</u>

Reminder: goal for this year:

Be a fit lean size to fit the black size six bathing suit I bought a few years back. I want to look good in it by July 1st and wear it through the summer.

9:30 p.m. I feel very blessed for another day of deliverance from overeating.

January 23, 2009

I'm very grateful for another day of deliverance from overeating and another day of exercising my body. I feel good when I take care of my body and I am visualizing myself lying on the Sandpoint beach in my black size six suit looking like I belong in it.

January 26, 2009

Last week of January—hurrah! I feel so good having had three weeks of deliverance from overeating. Hoorah! I feel so much better, happier, smarter, prettier, more energetic, and more confident. Please help me remember Lord how crappy it feels to eat crap and to overeat.

Remember Ruth, remember.

February also came and went with more prayers and workouts.

February 6, 2009

Last night I tried a higher level video workout—58 minutes. To me it was very high intensity. I almost passed out. Good workout. I continue to be grateful for deliverance from overeating and for continuing my good workout schedule.
I feel healthy and fit and I know my size is going down. I can tell by the way my clothes fit.

February 12, 2009

Today Alicia told me my butt looks smaller than a few weeks ago. My regular workouts are helping.

March 4, 2009

I feel good about my fitness level and have had two months now of moderation in eating and exercising and I am noticing the results in the way my clothes fit.

Spring came again and with it came continuing momentum in the fight against fat.

May 18, 2009

I've had a very physically active day—70 minute walk this morning then I mowed the lawn (two hours.), then I had a nap then went for a two hour bike ride. Tonight I did my DVD workout without the lower body exercises—the bike ride covered for that.

# The seven deadly sugars

If life were never stressful, I wouldn't need to diet or to binge. Momentum came crashing down again with the ever changing events in my life.

May 27, 2009

I've been out to a retirement barbecue. I'm not sure why I feel so awkward at social events. I kind of got carried away eating desserts. Ugh. Now I feel stuffed. I guess I felt anxious being around others in a social setting.

May 28, 2009

Ugh, now I remember the awfulness of overeating and the morning after blahs that come with it. Now I know why moderation in eating is a much happier route to follow.

In June 2009 my former husband was in a serious car crash and miraculously survived. I mention it here because it seemed to somehow be a catalyst for me to spin into weeks of food hell and self-hatred for whatever reason.

June 7, 2009

Alicia had a birthday sleepover on Friday with seven friends, lots of pizza, junk food, and ice cream cake. I had some ice cream cake.

I'm not sure why I'm feeling so down on myself and thinking of all my faults and flaws and failures in marriage. It seems to be that my former husband's crash has triggered a lot of remorse, regret, and guilt in me. It could also be that I've had too much sugar and junk food lately and my glycemic index is stressed. I really don't like dwelling on negative traits.

June 30, 2009

I seem to have descended once again into sugar hell. First I have the illusion that I can eat a little and get away with it, and then I seem to eat more and more. I feel troubled, anxious, scared, and all those negative emotions that go along with eating junk—poor sleeping, low energy, and so forth.

When I'm tired I feel very low and tend to eat sugar and crap. It's a bad cycle to be caught in.

Here are all the icky reasons not to eat sugar and all refined carbs:

- depression
- hot sweats
- anxiety, worry, and then I start fretting over money. Ugh. I hate getting into money worries
- bloating, gas, constipation
- fatigue, not to mention weight gain. I can feel it creeping back on—actually piling rather than creeping.

It was time to bring back compulsive exercising to combat the compulsive eating. From one extreme to the other, I teetered on the edge of insanity. You gotta love extremists! I was a terrorist to my own body and soul.

July 1, 2009

Today was my flush out day after several days of too much sugar and junk, so I started the day with a ninety minute hike with my neighbor then followed immediately with a full body weighted workout for sixty minutes.

My breakfast was raw berries, after which I went to the grocery store to stock up on fresh fruit for my flush out fruit day. After eating a pile of fresh blueberries, strawberries, cantaloupe, mango, and banana I set out for an extended bike ride through the country side. This lasted about three hours and by the time I pushed my bike the last leg up my very long and tortuous hill to home I was very exhausted. It was time for a nap and more fruit. Then this evening I walked another hour to attend my food addict meeting. No one showed up. After a few bitter thoughts I hiked back home again and watered my garden.

I am now feeling flushed out and physically exhausted and ready to go to bed. Fitness feels so much better than fatness. There is no food high comparable to the high of exercise. What a great way to celebrate Canada Day.

# Blah blah blog

In the summer of 2009 I started writing a blog about fitness and weight loss. A number of these entries are included in my journaling. It is clear to see when I was on the high of losing weight and when I switched to the lows of gaining weight. My introduction to this blog was cautiously optimistic about my relationship with food and my body.

July, 2009

I am a middle aged chronic dieter who has, through a twelve-step program and exercise, managed to find peace with my body most days. Exercise is my therapy and the ultimate mood elevator. Someday when I have the time I would like to be a compulsive exerciser rather than compulsive eater.

July 8, 2009

Today I read a quotation from a long time sober alcoholic. It was something like, 'my worst days in recovery were still better than my best days binging'.

As a long time food binger and dieter, I can attest to his sentiment that yes, my worst days of abstinence from compulsive overeating are better than my best days of binging.

I have had a lovely hike up the mountain and I've done an hour of full body weights. Now I'm soaking in the tub and feeling my muscles burning calories. No amount of food of any taste, or of any brand, has ever felt as good as this.

July 10, 2009

It's amazing how one simple change in behavior can have such a tremendous impact on every aspect of my life. Since adding weighted workouts in January this year to my fitness regime I feel much more confident and powerful. Not just physically, but spiritually, intellectually, emotionally and even socially. There seems to be so much wisdom and power built into the cells of the body and exercise seems to unleash that power and wisdom.

As I sweat through my weighted workout this morning, I couldn't help think of the first few days in January when the skies were grey and my holiday binge was weighing heavily on my butt and thighs. How gloomy I felt and yet I knew that by small and simple things are great things brought to pass. Just simply doing that weighted workout consistently the past six months has fuelled such a positive and optimistic drive in me, not to mention chiseling off the holiday binge. Just yesterday my neighbor and walking buddy commented that she sees a big difference in the backs of my arms and how much more muscular they are.

July 12, 2009

As I drove by the ice-cream place today a sign caught my eye: tin roof sundae blizzards. My heart started racing and for one fleeting moment I believed that blizzard was just what I wanted and needed on a hot summer day. The loud voice that hates me was trying hard to convince me with such arguments as, 'Oh come on its summer.' and, 'You live only once.' and 'You've got to have some pleasure in life.' and on and on. Then the little voice that loves me said, 'Sugar never was happiness.' I believed the little voice because it loves me and I know it is true. Sugar is not life nor happiness nor summer. If I live only once let that life be filled with health and vitality not self-imposed illness and misery.

July 14, 2009

Someone once said that our bodies are apt to be our autobiographies. I would like to add that our bodies speak volumes about our attitudes toward ourselves and toward life in general. I have observed several body biographies in my world this week. There are bodies that say, 'I hate myself'. Some of these bodies use their weight to intimidate and control others. They are not satisfied within themselves and clearly demonstrate this in their rudeness to coworkers, family members, and strangers alike. Not only are they physically uncomfortable in their own skin but emotionally and socially uncomfortable as well. It's as if they are attempting to assert power through size rather than through positive esteem of self and others. What they lack in emotional and social size they are attempting to make up in physical size. Sadly no amount of physical size can compensate for a shrivelled and starving mind and soul. No amount of food can compensate for failure to feed the soul.

# Have diet will travel

During the summer of 2009 I was occupied collecting and analyzing data for my doctoral dissertation. I also travelled to India to watch my son play for Team Canada in the world volleyball championships. It was a rather spontaneous crazy move prompted by the carefree spontaneity of my daughter, Alicia. Some entries make reference to this trip and the experiences there. I was thankfully relatively slim for me (hovering around 150 pounds, which by all accounts is not slim for a 5'4" woman, but slim for me at the time).

<u>July 15, 2009</u>

Yesterday after work I popped into a local dress shop to look for India-appropriate clothing (i.e. loose and cool) for my upcoming trip to the world championships of volleyball. Upon entering the store the first thing that caught my eye of course was the Mumu-style big dresses that have no form. As I fondly fingered the first formless dress, my daughter's voice came to me saying, 'Mom, if it looks fat on the rack it's going to look fat on you. You're not big so quit buying big formless clothes.' I listened to her direction and went deeper into the dress shop finding the perfect dress, a smocked fitted bodice and long flowing skirt. It was a match made in heaven. I knew I had to have it even before looking at the price tag. It was off the rack and into my arms and off to the checkout confidently knowing that this was a compliment to my appearance rather than a detriment. I was reminded however, of how hard those old habits are to change—big baggy clothes seem to have been my comfort and norm for many years. Exactly why that is I don't know. Perhaps a deep seated belief that I needed to be hidden—that I couldn't really be who I am. A huge part of being healthy in mind, body, and spirit is allowing me to be who I am as well as allowing others to see who I am and to know me.

July 19, 2009

Last night I attended a benefit dinner and silent auction. As I perused the silent auction items my attention fell on a basket of dark chocolate promising stress free and effortless weight loss. My heart started pounding erratically and visions of being size six by Monday danced through my head. For one fleeting moment of euphoria I was sucked in and stopped to read the fine print. Somewhere between 'all natural' and 'energy', my left brain rationality kicked in and reminded me of my previous experience with the magic weight loss chocolate. Back in the winter one of my students supplied me with some dark chocolate claiming magical weight loss powers. The package was dropped off in broad daylight in a public place so I naturally thought it was above board and I didn't promise her better grades because of it so I felt pure about the whole thing.

Okay, now before you pass judgement on me, think, who wouldn't want to eat chocolate that boasted of magical transformative powers? Just the promise of boosting metabolic rate and suppressing appetite while eating dark chocolate wafers gave me a dopamine rush. It sure beats the hell out of okra and kale (aka grass and slime). I had visions of not only being size six in time for Valentine's Day, but also of being taller, prettier, younger, friendlier, and smarter—not to mention that my teeth would be whiter and George Clooney would return my call—all this from eating that magic dark chocolate.

Well it didn't take long to have my fantastical visions shattered. I was on a 'trip' of sorts, the likes of which I had never experienced. I was jumpy, moody, paranoid, and grouchy, besides feeling like a hill of polygamous formica ants had taken up residence in my liver (and yes I DO know that formica ants live polygamously—I learned that in my dissertation literature search). Suddenly the 'too good to be true' magic chocolate had fallen from grace and I was back to reality, a wiser yet no thinner woman. I didn't bid on the silent auction chocolate.

July 22, 2009

I just got in from a refreshing swim in the neighbor's fish pond. As the fish swam around me threatening to nibble at my toes, I secretly fantasized about them performing liposuction on my butt and thighs. If I could just stay in the pond long enough I might emerge actually fitting into the size six bathing suit I insisted on stuffing myself into. Hey, I can have my dreams right? Don't the gurus (whoever the gurus are) say if you can see it you can be it? I'm not sure that this includes seeing fish suck the cellulite off my thighs or not, but it's my fantasy and I'm sticking to it. If you're going to fantasize it might as well be good. I never could understand people daydreaming about all the bad things that could happen (although I must confess at times allowing this destructive habit to destroy my peace). It just seems that if you're going to think and imagine, why not think and imagine positive, happy, hopeful images? I read somewhere that if we knew how powerful our thoughts are, we would never again think another negative thought. Even the Bible says, 'as a man thinketh in his heart so is he,' and I'm sure that goes for women too. I don't know about you but I'm not about to denounce the Bible. After all, it is the Bible! Who'd have thought that the SECRET wasn't a secret after all? It was in the Bible all these millennia. Think lean, think strong, think size six (okay, okay, so I AM a dress size, and a bathing suit size, and a pant size).

July 23, 2009

Over 2000 years ago, Hippocrates, the very father of medicine, recommended diet and exercise rather than drugs. Somewhere in the last two millennia his sage wisdom has been supplanted with the money-motivated pharmaceutical and fast food companies. We need a return to the wisdom of the ages—a return to whole food and exercise to heal the ills that plague prosperous nations. It has been said that the number one health problem outside North America is starvation and the number one health problem inside North America is obesity. It is no wonder then that it is man-made diseases, not mysterious super-bugs that are killing Americans. It's no surprise to me that one day working in the ER a doctor looked out at the overflowing waiting room and said, 'I can tell you what's wrong with everyone out there without even seeing them—they eat too much!' I hate to admit it, but he was right. So many ills, aches, pains, stressed joints, and failing hearts are directly linked to or exacerbated by obesity. We don't need a pill; we need a push off the couch. Is it time to go back to the sage wisdom of Hippocrates and admit that more than two millennia later he was in fact right?

July 24, 2009

Isn't it amazing what a number on the scale can do to the start of the day? For over a year I refused to stand on the scale but I started this addictive ritual once again this past month. Now I ask, wasn't it enough to have clothes fitting that used to not fit, to have them loose and comfortable where once they were binding like debt? To have people stop me at the grocery store and tell me I look like a rail (yes, I kid you not, she said a rail!)? NO, that just wasn't enough—the lure of those magic numbers on the scale seemed to beckon with greater force than chocolate during a PMS storm. Like many a PMS storm I succumbed to the lure of the scale, only to be thrown into a fit of misery because the numbers, those magic numbers, weren't as low as I had anticipated. All of a sudden the pleasure of feeling lean and fit was sacrificed to the scale gods and their numbers. What is SO important about quantifying everything? Wasn't it Einstein that said, 'Not everything that counts can be counted and not everything that can be counted counts?'

Anyways, back to my scale woes. One year I taped '130' over the digital weight display on my scale. I had read somewhere that if I saw that number every morning when I weighed then my mind would turn my body into that weight. I think it was working until my 6'4" hulk of a fireman son was visiting and removed it—seems he didn't want to weigh 130 pounds. Go figure! That was two years ago at Christmas and I have no idea why I never replaced the magic number back on my scale. Maybe that's why it didn't work. After all these decades of cyclic and frenzied dieting and having my moods dictated by the scale (if the numbers are up, my mood is down, if the numbers are down, my mood is up) you'd think that I could get over it, but no. Here I am in my 50s still being ruled by the numbers on a scale. Not only am I a dress size, I seem to be a number on the scale too.

July 26, 2009

As I've been packing for India, 'pack lightly' seems to come to mind. Travel will be so much easier if I take along only the actual essentials. Not only is travel made easier but life as well by packing lightly and leaving unnecessary baggage where it belongs. Emotional baggage is often reflected in one's physical countenance. Just as dragging heavy baggage on a long journey weighs me down and slows my progress, so also does dragging the grudges, hurts, resentments, and guilt from the past weigh down my soul and slow my progress in the journey of life. I do not have to carry the past forever planted on my hips and thighs and etched into the misery lines on my face. Just as I can remove excess baggage from my travel bags I can also let go of the disappointments, mistakes, and sorrows of the past and move forward with a perfect brightness of hope into a future that is filled only with exalting experiences. I've heard that the Buddhists say attachment is the greatest form of self-cruelty. I believe this to be true especially with attachments to the miseries and mistakes of the past.

# What you gain in India stays in India

This next entry reveals that my eating frenzy was far from cured. Just because the breakfast buffet was free, and just because it was enormous, I ate and ate volumes, convincing myself that it was okay because it was, after all, nutritious. I looked at what others in the restaurant ate, noting their consumption was much smaller than mine and wondering why I could eat so much food. They probably thought the same thing. But it's FREE, DUH!

August 7, 2009

The breakfast buffet here is delicious. I usually eat a large breakfast—fresh papaya, pineapple, melons, some bran cereal with nuts, date, prunes—then have bacon, sausage, and some Indian dishes usually beans, rice, and lentils. I am getting lots of fiber. Some days I haven't eaten a second meal. Some days we've had Domino's pizza at the games. I have enjoyed using the fitness center and pool daily. I hope I'm keeping up my muscle fitness.

After my trip to India I returned home with maxed-out credit cards and no permanent job. My college contract had once again ended for another term. It was a fat wreck waiting to happen.

## August 21, 2009

My anxieties over money are returning as I face the next few months without permanent work and also face maxed out credit cards from my trip to India, education, and kid expenses. As has been my habit in the past, my insecurities have driven me to food for comfort rather than turning me to God. Today I will refocus on God rather than food.

Today an old friend was visiting. We had a good walk and talk. She came over for supper. I made lasagna, Greek salad, spaghetti squash, and apple crisp. I ate too much.

## August 22, 2009

The other night I had a visit from the ghosts of wardrobes past. For some reason I was pondering my clothing sizes and it dawned on me that much of what I have worn most of my life was either too big or too small. I'm not sure if this had some deeper meaning or association with my inability, perhaps to accept myself as I am. Some experts have opined that self-acceptance is the beginning of positive change, whether that be physical or psychological. It seems rather contradictory that when I accept myself as I am, I will then have access to the powers that promote change. I don't have to dress bigger or smaller to hide what I am. It's okay to be what I am right now. Whatever size that is, I will look and feel better if it fits than if it doesn't. For the ghost of today I promise to be what I am, where I am, and who I am. Just for today I am wearing clothes that fit.

Despite the self pep talk, I could not quite come to grips with the anxiety and eating monster.

<u>August 22, 2009</u>

I am feeling anxious and starting to eat junk food compulsively. Help!

## Herd mentality eating

Once again my house was full of family and friends coming and going. Not that I minded this. I love my family. I just seem to eat more when they're around. It's the eating with the herd mentality. My son and his volleyball colleague were staying while doing a volleyball camp. My sister was visiting and with her visits came wonderful feasts with other family coming over. Fun for sure, but also very fattening for me.

<u>September 6, 2009</u>

My sister was visiting this past week. She was cooking and baking here. She has made some delectable desserts every day and we've had family over to share in them.
I haven't been sleeping well all week, probably the flood of too many rich desserts upsetting my body chemistry. This week my behavior has reaffirmed to me that I am indeed powerless over my addiction and I need the power of God in my life daily—no, hourly and minutely.

The excess of summer gave way to the inevitable misery of weight gain. The family and friends left but alas, the fat did not. It settled heavily on my butt and thighs. My baby entered her last year of high school and my older daughter visited with some rather shocking though exciting news.

September 8, 2009

So now the summer vacation in food Babylon is officially done.

September 15, 2009

Always expect the unexpected. That was my mantra for this past week of surprises in my life. When my daughter announced that she was planning a wedding for a month from now, I felt a sense of panic. Not panic induced by wondering if this is the right decision for her; and not panic for the amount it may cost me; and not panic for the fact that she is marrying someone I have yet to meet. No—my panic was fuelled by my weight fixation. How much weight can I lose in a month? What style of dress will make me look thinnest and will I look like a fifty something fat mother of the bride? I know! It's sick really that amidst all the excitement and hype of her starting a journey with a man who will love and cherish her, I am obsessing about my weight. The stress is enough to send me plunging head first into a tub of ice-cream (sugar free of course). Obviously there is still some room for improvement in my psychological health.
When all else fails, jump into the cabbage soup diet. Lucky for me a gardening friend dumped some fresh cabbage on me just this week. It was a sign; absolutely providential. I am meant to be on the cabbage soup diet for the week leading up to my daughter's wedding. How can a chronic dieter resist the temptation? Just in time to squeeze myself respectably into my mother of the bride outfit.

# Fat expansion

I did manage to squeeze into that size ten brown suit for the wedding and it fit me exactly long enough to get through the ceremony and dinner. From there it was all uphill on the scale as I ate myself into another fat frenzy.

October 12, 2009

Thanksgiving Day. I am taking the time to list my gratitude prayer to God. He understands me. So my blessings that I thank God for as they free flow into my mind.
Healthy body and my skirt didn't split at the wedding.

October 16, 2009

This past week I have transitioned from being a mother to being a mother in law. The week leading up to this wonderful event saw me cabbage soup dieting in anticipation of fitting into my suit. The week following this blessed event has seen me bread and cheese dieting to assuage the anxieties and uncertainties that often accompany threats to familiarity. If my lovely daughter's wedding was the only change blessing my life at present I may not be feeling such anxiety. However, I returned home to see my dear neighbor and walking buddy packing up to move to a distant city and the weather definitely transitioned from Indian summer to outright prairie-like winter. To top it off I turned 54. How the hell did that happen? I could have sworn I was just eighteen yesterday!

For some unknown reason, and I'm sure someday I will have a psychobiological explanation for it, food seems to provide the illusion of security and comfort when the world around me is seemingly spinning out of control. Hence the bread and cheese. Lots of it. And with it the illusion of home and family, love and comfort, security and peace. Life may be changing and the years flying by, but bread and cheese is still bread and cheese.

November 4, 2009

What is it with us and our pig-out holidays? Having just come through Halloween, I wonder what the hell anything has to do with chocolate and yet every holiday that comes along seems to require chocolate or it hasn't been properly observed and celebrated. After taking my lovely daughter and her charming husband to the Spokane airport, I did some respectable grocery shopping at Costco – no junk food or anything chocolate related (okay, so I ate the free Costco samples and some of them were less than virtuous). I abstained from purchasing junk food until I was almost home then the panic hit. What if my friend brings her five children trick or treating to my house tonight and I don't have anything to give them except a carrot? Not that there's anything wrong with a carrot. So I pulled over to the gas station and convenience store to buy junk food to hand out. Of course no one came trick or treating and guess who ate the treats? I'm not even going to go there. All because of some pagan ridiculous holiday that never had anything to do with food until the capitalistic pigs decided there was money to be made. Along with millions of others, I chose to buy and eat into it. I wonder if I could swing the trends and start cabbage soup for all holidays. Doesn't that sound like something worth celebrating?

# Shoot me up with fat vaccine

<u>November 5, 2009</u>

This week I finally gave into the vaccine hounds and got flu vaccines. Two: one for the regular flu and one for the H1N1, commonly known on the streets as swine flu. To tell you the truth I would rather have been vaccinated against pig-out flu. H1N1 could stand for heavy one/no one. To a food junkie and one who suffers from pigging out, the swine flu could mean binging sickness. My mind got racing and fantasizing about a vaccine against pigging out and becoming fat. Now THERE'S a vaccine I would like to be known for. Can you imagine what it would be like if there was a simple shot you could take that would prevent you from eating too much? I would be laughing all the way to the scale. Of course there would be some industries that would fight its release and availability to the masses, like for instance the food industry. Wouldn't that cut into their profits if people were getting a shot to stop them from overeating? What about the weight loss industry? Wouldn't they be ticked if everyone finally solved their weight problems? Whatever would Jenny Craig, Nutrisystem, and Weight Watchers do? What about the plus size fashions and all those styles and clothes designed to make us look thinner? There they go right out the syringe with the pig-out flu.

# Time flies when you're gaining weight

November 18, 2009

This past week I've been poring over my old journals preparing my dissertation—a veritable stroll down memory lane. What shocks me most about these journals is the continual theme of having difficulty with controlling sugar intake. One journal when I was in my early 20s talks about me reading a book on the health hazards of sugar and how I vowed to cut it out of my life for good. Other journal entries throughout the years have the same theme, mostly bemoaning my overindulgence in sugar laden foods and the day after with its unpleasant hangover symptoms—headache, lethargy, depression and so forth. I note that there are no entries discussing any problem with controlling broccoli or onion intake. I even have one entry that vows to conquer the problem so I won't have to deal with it in my 40s. Of course back then I didn't think I would ever be forty. So here I am, thirty years later, bemoaning a problem that I clearly identified in writing while still in my youth. When I write my autobiography it will certainly have to be titled, 'Time Flies When You're Eating Sugar,' or how about, 'Time

Flies When You're Gaining Weight,' or maybe just, 'Time Flies'.

# In and out of the binge tank

As the binging persisted and I looked longingly at that brown suit that no longer fit, cabbage soup dieting once again sucked me in, if only for a moment.

November, 2009

I started a cabbage soup diet yesterday to once again purge my excesses with sugar. I've been reading past journals and see years and years of food problems and trying to stop sugar. Here I am at 54 with this same old problem. Isn't that pathetic?

Other stress factors in my life included the loss of my dear friend and walking buddy (my shrink in more ways than one), the loss of steady work, the loss of summer, the loss of daylight, and loss of so much. But sadly, not weight. Then I had the return to shift work. Ugh, here comes the night shift again.

November 26, 2009

Something about night shift flips my whole system on its head and with it any sense of orderliness with eating and exercise. Having come off a twelve hour night shift this morning, I am feeling the effects of night shift hangover complete with a confused body and mind. I'm not sure exactly what it is about sugar and salty snacks that seem to pass the perils of night shift. I suppose there's a false sense that they are giving comfort to replace the comfort of sleep. Or perhaps they give the sense that I am avoiding the pain of night shift by filling it with the perceived pleasure of food or perhaps my concern for health is shot all to hell by the effects of sleep deprivation. Whatever it is, I am grateful that my body is hurting. It's a painful reminder of why I don't want refined carbs in my body. I wonder how many times this can happen before I actually commit to abstinence from sugar. AA says that when the pain of the habit is greater than the pain of change then change occurs. Tonight the pain of the habit is forefront (literally) in my mind as I suffer one of those frontal, distal, and global headaches that only sugar can elicit. How can the pleasure of something so sweet give birth to the experience of so much suffering? I guess I will add this to my list of questions for God. Until then, I remain a mortal suffering from the effects of the fridge.

November 28, 2009

I am suffering a residual headache from another sugar binge. Ugh! I am making cookies for Alicia's volleyball fundraiser and eating smarties and chocolate chips and donuts at work then Pepsi to stay awake on night shift. My poor body, it is suffering so much.

# Fat lamentations

As the nights got longer, my butt and belly and binge feasts got bigger while the light in my soul shrunk to a faint glimmer.

<u>December 14, 2009</u>

Its 4:30 a.m. and I have been lying awake for about two hours now, suffering from the effects of yet again another feeding binge and pondering on my powerlessness over my addiction and why, why, why, I find myself still suffering from sugar overdose. Why do I have this problem that I seem to beat in spurts only to have it resurface to haunt me? I feel gross. Too much sugar basically and clothes that are all tight again.

I have been praying to have this weakness become strong unto me. I know that when I commit to abstinence from sugar and junk food my life is much more serene and peaceful but for some reason I slip and fall into the food hell again; the swine returning to her wallowing in the mud pie.

My focus is completely gone and I am lost to the power of the addiction. I have to constantly refocus on the simple principles of the program. I need to get back to step one admitting that I am powerless over my addiction, believing that the power of God can restore me to sanity.

Yesterday I attended a church Christmas dinner. I had been asked to give a ten minute talk after the meal so I had prepared a Christmas message, which I thoroughly enjoyed writing. Unfortunately I limited the spiritual experience for myself by excessively indulging my carnal desires with desserts. I have been feeling the tension of sugar and worry and excess building the past couple months and have failed to get a grip on it. I suppose the problem is largely lack of commitment and feeling insecure and tossed about by the uncertainties and moods of each day as it comes.

Why did I allow myself to just give in to the excess and eat and eat and eat? It starts a terrible cascade of excess that seems to take months to recover from. Perhaps assertiveness is a problem. I need to speak up for myself and make my desires known. It's okay not to indulge when others are.

Then it was a cabbage soup diet to get ready for Joan's wedding. I fit the new suit just long enough to get through the wedding and pictures and it hasn't fit since and it's such a nice suit and I looked so good in it. I wanted so badly (not badly enough) to be able to fit that suit and wear it to church but alas it has not happened. The suit hangs in my closet waiting for me to get myself back on the program of abstinence and off the roller coaster of binging and purging.

Where did I go? Where did that serene, determined, committed, abstinent person go, the one who wanted so much to conquer food hell; the one who wanted health and vitality above sugar and misery? It seems that the fall starts with a simple taste then ends up in the depths of sugar hell.

So how can I turn this around now and not wait 'til New Year's Day to get back on recovery road, the straight and narrow path that leads to serenity and sanity rather than anxiety and misery?

November was a lean month financially (too bad it wasn't a lean month as far as food goes). I need to face my fears about my finances. I guess I knew it would come to this eventually given that I have been spending a lot on education which I don't regret. Exactly what I think eating will do to assuage these doubts and fears, I do not know. I guess I feel like maybe I deserve misery and being fat and bloated and poor. I really don't know what is at the base of this insane behavior.

So here I am coming to the close of another year still fighting the demons that have plagued me for decades. Though I am not quite as fat as I was a year ago, I am heading that way and if I don't head off this path I will be bloated up again to that size. It's ridiculously embarrassing after decades of ups and downs and ups and downs and ups and downs again.

What the hell is the matter with me? Why can't I conquer this once and for all, Lord? Why can't I conquer this? Why do I allow that first bite of sugar and believe that it will not hurt anything? Why am I deceived over and over and over again and give into the desire to eat? Why can I not stay converted to a sugar free life knowing what havoc it wreaks with my mind, body, emotions, and spirit? For me it is a deadly drug that takes me into a fit of despair and depression and doubt and fear, worry, and self-loathing.

December 18, 2009

It seems as I get older I am much more sensitive to the nuances in my physical reactions to food. I love being free from compulsive eating. It is a one-way rapid transit to misery, depression, despair, despondency, self-loathing, and of course obesity and cellulite. The opposite is serenity, joy, peace, esteem, confidence, and love for self and others.

The demons won. The year closed as it had opened, with me fat, fearful, and compulsively filling myself with food.

# Cry me a pizza

My fears over my daughter becoming an adult seemed to consume a lot of my energy. I'm not sure what I thought food was going to do. Maybe, like Neil Diamond's *Red Red Wine*, I hoped it would go to my head and help me forget that change was closing in on me. Instead of going to my head, it went straight to my hips and thighs and belly—and I didn't forget a damn thing!

December 24, 2009 3:00 a.m.

I feel like an idiot. Here I am once again suffering from the effects of excess food—mainly sugar and fat. What the heck is my problem and why does it keep coming up over and over and over again? I am basically in the same spot I was last year this time.

Here I am doing the same thing over and over and over again. I am awake with a rumbling gut; my suffering digestive system has to work overtime to process my excess late night eating of ice-cream and cookies.

So why do I eat to excess? I guess I get that arrogant 'who cares' attitude and let my prideful carnal nature take over. Before I know it I am eating uncontrollably like a zombie that can't stop. Last night I just ate and ate and ate, even though I was tired and should have just gone to bed. I was alone and could have peacefully read my way to sleep.

Am I a fraud? I feel the pressure and humiliation of once again gaining weight. I hate that. I hate it when I have been losing weight, feeling great with food and exercise and getting compliments from others then I cave into the carnal cravings of my body and start gaining once again. I feel like an idiot; I feel humiliated; I feel like a failure and a loser who just can't get her act together for any length of time.

I guess this recycled failure at managing food and weight is downright humiliating and I feel like I am a hypocrite because I am not living what I am preaching. I love the abstinent active lifestyle free of sugar and junk food, and yet here I am smack dab in the middle of the very lifestyle I decry and disdain. Hypocrisy is screaming loud and clear. I don't want to be a hypocrite. I hate it when people use stress as their excuse for everything, but I must admit that I feel stressed.

I have been battling my stupid weight problem my whole adult life and here it still is.

So what would my perfect 2010 wish look like?

My wish list for 2010: [not all inclusive]

1. Abstinence from compulsive eating.

# Effects of the fall

So now here I am in to 2010 and still trying to catch that elusive victory over the flesh.

January 1, 2010

The Greek philosopher Democritus is credited with having said, "Throw moderation to the winds and the greatest pleasures bring the greatest pains." My own personal experience supports this claim. Having just come through that most excessive of all excesses of holidays, Christmas, the presence of the pain of excess is almost as abundant as the snow that has been falling all day. From shortbread to monster cookies to turkey and stuffing there has been no food moderation in my house for a number of weeks. The pleasure of excess has now turned into the pain of consequences—a few more rolls and cellulite that are now the focus of once again working out one day at a time. It's January once again and moderation is the word of the month.

The magic of the New Year and its transformative powers seemed to elude me. I was left confused, fat, and medicating myself with more food.

Only weeks into the New Year I fell while walking in the snow and broke my arm. This put an abrupt stop to my weight workouts, which I was convinced, were going to get me back on track with food management. My legs still worked, but something totally flipped me out about exercise after that fall. Likely it was just an excuse, not only to stop weights, but to medicate myself with food. My all-or-nothing monster was screaming at me and I succumbed to the pressure.

February 12, 2010

I continue to struggle with my carnal self. As I have been pondering this I sometimes feel like I am being selfish by asking God to help me overcome such a seemingly stupid and insignificant thing as overeating. Then it dawned on me that it isn't such a selfish thing because neglect of self usually means neglect of others. Health in all domains hinges on health in the physical domain. I need my body and I need it to be healthy in order to serve and to have health, emotionally, spiritually, socially, and so forth. So it really isn't a selfish thing to ask for God's help in caring for my body. Yet I seem to continue such negative patterns.

Yesterday there were blueberry muffins at work. All white flour of course and basically void of nutrition, but I indulged not only in one but four, then I felt bloated.

# Soul food versus sick food

February 15, 2010

I am amazed at what a difference in my life feeding my body nutritiously makes for my emotional health. When I don't eat sugar and junk food I feel so much more peaceful and confident. Anxiety and fear seem to leave me, and hope and optimism return. What a blessing that is! Please remind me Lord of this, next time I think I just have to have whatever that available poison is in the staff room, or at a social or whatever holiday I think is associated with chocolate or cookies or pastries or whatever. There really is no peace or joy in junk food. The peace and joy come from a body that is nurtured with the fruits of the earth just as the spirit is nurtured with the fruits of the Spirit, and not the physical 'spirits' we mortals use as a crutch for lacking God in our lives.

February 19, 2010

Somehow that reminder didn't keep me from excess eating yesterday when I attended the college professional development day in Cranbrook with other Creston faculty. I was okay until after the session when we visited a former faculty who now lives there and he and his wife had a table full of goodies for us. I did not know we would be there for so long (almost three hours) and I felt my plans for the day were altered, so I guess the moment and the change and the social anxiety all contributed to my over indulging. To begin with I was hungry since it had been four hours since I ate lunch, but after the initial hunger was satisfied I continued eating because of taste and sugar trigger and it seemed to facilitate socializing. So I went to bed full and fatigued and mildly disappointed with the sessions of the day.

Anyway, I woke up feeling bloated and a bit headachy so I am suffering the effects of my fall into sugar again. I am going to speedily forgive myself and move forward rather than beat myself up all day which will only make me want to eat all day too.

February 20, 2010

I find it difficult to manage eating when I am away at volleyball tournaments. I want to get my eating back to abstinence from overeating and junk food. I want to get a program going again so that I can be back to a more enjoyable fitness level when I embark on my post mothering life.

I know that I cannot reach my potential as long as my food demons are ruling me.

February 25, 2010

The tournament passed successfully with Alicia's team winning all their games and coming home with the gold medal. Another long and tiring drive and I seem to be suffering with fatigue and insomnia this week for some reason—partly because of my food excesses.

I think that I need to just forget about the problem and focus on developing talents and drawing near to God.

# The James factor

My daughter and her husband were visiting during the late winter awaiting the birth of their son, who arrived on March 8th. So for a time I had extra family and a newborn in the house.

March 23, 2010

The other day I had an epiphany while cuddling my restless little grandson. He had recently breast fed but like most newborns was continuing to frantically search for something to put in his mouth. As I attempted to sooth his panic at not having anything in his mouth, I said, "Okay little James, you don't need to have something in your mouth constantly to be happy". Then came the epiphany—with his little eyes focusing on my face I felt like he was responding, "and neither do you Grandma!" (Of course I was stuffing MY face at the time!). Was the universe sending me a message or what? Out of the mouths of babes comes indescribable wisdom. That epiphany fills my soul as I continue my journey to wholeness. Days after sharing this experience with a walking buddy, she too said that it continued to be in her thoughts whenever she reached for something to put into her mouth. She calls it the "James Factor". Go James!

I've heard it said that knowledge is power. I have learned a fair amount about nutrition and addiction for some time and yet I seem to lack power. I believe a more appropriate statement would be that God is power. The application of knowledge provides access to the power of God. So it appears that knowledge does have a huge role to play in providing the power to effect change. Knowledge was all around me and yet, no power to overcome. My junk food cravings made me the real junkie.

March, 2010

Last night I saw on the CTV news that researchers have now discovered that junk food is as addictive as cocaine and heroin (like I needed a researcher to tell me that!). Particularly for those sensitive to sugar, the addictive cravings are equal to cocaine and heroin addicts. No wonder I get anxious every time I get near sugar. I wonder what the odds are of having it illegalized. Would this help those sugar sensitive souls like myself? It's back to recovery for me, at least just for today.

March 30, 2010 4:40 a.m.

How many times must I go through this insomniac eating routine? Last night there was a story on the news about the addictive nature of junk food, particularly sugar. I have intuitively known this for forty years in myself and yet I still struggle. What's wrong with me? Why can't I stop this?

April 9, 2010

As a teenager in 4-H clubs I learned the motto learn to do by doing. I could alter this motto to say learn to think by doing. Much has been said about the power of thought to effect action; however, the flip side of this equation is that action also influences thought. Take the action of eating salt, fat, and sugar, which stimulates the pleasure centers of my brain, starting a chain reaction of thinking that influences my brain to think of salt, fat, and sugar. The more I eat, the more my brain thinks about eating and tells me to go for these substances. On the other hand, eating nutritious food influences my brain to stimulate thoughts of eating nutritious food. The more I eat nutritious food, the more I want nutritious food and thoughts of junk food gradually fade away. Not only am I what I eat, but what I eat creates what I think, which further influences what I eat.

It seemed that messages and signs were all around me but none of them internalized to transform my sinking soul from its downward spiral into the great and spacious abyss of food obsession.

April 13, 2010

The other day as I was walking to my doctor's appointment I was laboring over the issue of overeating. My walking chant was, "Why do I overeat? Why do I overeat?" When I got to my doctor's office I looked up to see on her magazine rack a cover story entitled, "Why we overeat". Epiphany strikes again. I was reminded of a number of sayings from Christian and other thoughts *ask and ye shall receive* and *when the student is ready, the teacher appears*. The magazine article led me to a book at the local library and more wisdom to win the war on junk food. The wisdom, of course, was what I have always known but needed some reinforcement again. For me the principle message was, when I eat food the way God created it, my body will look the way He created it.

April 20, 2010

For the past three weeks I have avoided all processed and packaged foods. Not only have I made the environment more beautiful, I have also created greater beauty in myself. My epiphany inspired by this simple act is that the more packaging of food that ends up as waste, the more of that packaged food will also end up on my waist. If it fills the landfill, it will fill my fat cells too. On the contrary, buying food that is not packaged or processed (i.e. real food, like raw fruits and vegetables, whole grains and beans, etc.) does not fill waste sites or my waist site. It's real food for me.

I am thankful now to have twenty days of abstinence from sugar and processed foods. What a difference this makes in my moods and how I feel about my body. Already I can feel the changing fat and energy levels. It is a blessing to once again have the gift of abstinence. I am committed to it. I have no desire for sugar or for junk food. I have only a desire for real food—wholesome whole food the way it was created. This is a tremendous blessing.

# Chewing what I bit off

Somewhere between the middle and end of May I once again derailed. Preparations were being made for my last child's graduation and I was feeling the pressure of a major transition coming up. I had also completed a PhD in psychology and it seemed that as the degrees of education went up so also did my weight, literally piled higher and deeper.

As determined as I was to not use food as my drug for transition, the power of the food habit was stronger than I was. Where did all my pep talks go in my time of need?

At this time I was also preparing for a faculty job interview in the States and planning to relocate in the hopes that I would be accepted to sing with the Mormon Tabernacle Choir. In preparation for this I was taking voice lessons, trying to sell my house, praying, fasting, and eating to avoid the fact that my last baby had become an adult.

May 31, 2010 Monday—3:30 a.m.

It is early morning and I am once again suffering the effects of sugar and eating before bed. I had the missionaries and some family over for dinner last night. After that I had the kitchen to clean up and then I ate some more cake and ice cream. I woke up thinking of Einstein's assertion that insanity is doing the same thing over and over again and expecting different results. Well what about the insanity of doing the same thing over and over again when you know the results will be the same and they won't be good? How insane is that? I suppose I am allowing the stress of trying to live too many days and too many lives at once get to me and increase my anxiety. I need to refocus on what is essential. Having God in my life is essential first and foremost. I wonder why I am here once again lying awake at night feeling restless and sick from eating. I am an intelligent woman so why do I do this over and over and over again?

This imbalance seems to be my weakness or thorn in the flesh. I need to go to the library and get some more books to read to keep focus on why I don't eat refined stuff, but I know in the back of my head I am thinking of Alicia's birthday tomorrow and how we want to get ice-cream cake. I love ice-cream. It is my favorite of all favorite treats. I wish I had a big waffle cone of pralines and cream or a mint Oreo blizzard or a big bowl of raspberries with vanilla ice-cream, and then I fantasize about the raspberries taking the fat out with their fiber and seeds. I feel reckless, like having a food bender and drowning myself in a vat of mud pie ice-cream. What is wrong with me or is there nothing wrong with me? If I could just run enough and do weights enough and hike enough and move doing anything enough, I could turn off this feeding frenzy and be svelte. But if not I can be beautiful anyway like my lovely voice teacher and her beautiful clothes and mannerisms.

# The proverbial fork in the road

June 5, 2010

It seems that whenever I see a fork in the road ahead I pick it up and eat (I DID say fork, didn't I). Anyway, I have some major decisions to make in my life in the next months and I am feeling the fork in the road syndrome and I'm eating in anticipation of the upcoming fork. Would life be easier then, with no choices to make? I heard a phrase once, "the freedom of no choice", asserting that sometimes simply having choices before us is stifling and imprisoning because of the overwhelming confusion it may cause, leading us to freeze in our tracks incapable of choosing. I am not advocating a life with no choices but sometimes it does seem that it would be easier to have only one choice for breakfast, one choice for lunch, and one choice for dinner with no alternatives in between. Not just food choices, but life choices as well. How little risk and anxiety there would be if I could see my path straight ahead of me for the next fifty years and know exactly what is going to happen, no unexpected forks or spoons or knives for that matter. For those of us who love to eat, a fork in the road is just that: a fork in the road.

June 19, 2010

I am enjoying my solitude for now. I need to meditate and get my strength back to get over my food binging of late. It's strange how the same problem keeps cropping up over and over and over again.

July 7, 2010

This past week I put my baby (eighteen year old baby that is) on the greyhound bus, off to another extended volleyball adventure. Something about seeing that greyhound bus drive away flipped me right into a tailspin of emptiness, feeling a sink hole deep in my mother heart. Before I knew it, and certainly before the bus was out of town, I found myself sitting in the DQ drive through with a large mint Oreo blizzard in my hand. Where did that come from? Perhaps it was my feeble attempt to fill the sink hole in my heart with ice-cream. Predictably the ice-cream didn't fill my empty heart but only the fat cells on my thighs. (My sister tells me she is taking out stock in DQ for this, my year of transition from emptying nest to emptied nest). A simple walk with a friend would have relieved the emptiness illusion much more effectively while strengthening rather than fattening my thighs. I could have bypassed the DQ and gone straight to the hills for a walk. Remember, remember, sugar never was happiness nor was it love, nor was it relief from any of life's challenges.

July 10, 2010 Saturday 3:45 a.m.

I have been lying awake for over an hour now. I started with being too hot then having to pee then debriefing my busy ER shift yesterday then on and on and on and on. Trying to force sleep is like trying to diet: the harder you try, the worse it gets. Now after reading the brain book I have, I am more concerned about getting enough sleep and that seems to just make things worse. Is this where a little knowledge is a bad thing? Now the birds are singing so I might as well stay awake and write.

<u>July 19, 2010</u>

I have had about 3 ½ hours of walking today. I should be a rake. Or at least not fat. Ah well. I am working on living for the day and stop worrying about weight.

# Fat faded glory

With the ending of another college contract my work life returned to shift work at the hospital. The summer was quickly fading and along with it all my grandiose plans for where I would be in 2010. By now I had planned to have sold my house, certified myself fat, and gone into a treatment center for food addicts, then to have landed a faculty job in some exciting university in the States. Above all I certainly was going to be slim. But there I was, a PhD graduate doing shift work as a general duty nurse, still pigging out on a regular basis, and still living large in Creston.

Something about Creston seemed to hold me and feed me and hold me and feed me and hold me and feed me. Someone told me once that it's the magnetic pull of the iron mountain range that keeps people here. For me it's more plausible that it's the pull of the mountains of abundant food produced annually all around and inside and outside of me. Regardless of the pull, there I was—still, there, still me.

> August 15, 2010
>
> My two night shifts were fairly quiet but left me eating continually.
>
> The other day I ran into a colleague that I haven't seen in awhile and was shocked to see her looking so lean,

healthy, and vibrant. When I commented on this, she said that she had lost fifty pounds in the past several months. Naturally the next question was, how? Like me she is one who has tried many diets and spent years going up and down the scale. This time she looked at the root of the problem rather than trying another band aid solution. As many of us chronic dieters know, food is not the problem; self-discipline is not the problem; desire is not the problem. So what is the problem? She, like me, was using food as a coping mechanism for stress, anxiety, fear, and so forth. After doing online counselling and identifying her food demons, she had begun to use food for what food is for—physical nourishment. I listened more intently as she shared what she had learned and how this learning had changed her view of food, dieting, weight, and stress. A key point in the plan was that all food fits when eaten in response to physical hunger. Our bodies have the wisdom to signal us when food is needed and to again signal when they have had enough. As I am learning and pondering these bites, I trust my body to tell me what it needs and when it needs it and how much it needs.

All food may fit, but all my clothes don't when I allow all food to fit. Some food just simply does not fit me. By late summer it was time to read another book in the hopes that it would be the one that would redeem me from the diet hell that had kept me trapped for so many years. Like the mice I had seen in previous traps, I too was sucked in by the lure of cheese and peanut butter and sugar and spice and everything twice or thrice.

## August 15, 2010

This week I am reading a book called *Women, Food, and God*. My sister loaned it to me. It's about emotional eating. I know that I am an emotional eater so just for today I am trying to eat for hunger only and not because I feel bad about not being invited to a friend's birthday; and not because I am feeling anxious about Alicia; and not because I am feeling alone and a failure at life; and not because I am feeling ashamed of my impulsive tongue; and not because I am alone.

There are many more things that are worse than being alone. For example, being alone AND fat!

# Empty nest, full stomach

Finally the great and dreadful day arrived when I launched my last of four children off to university in a distant city, well prepared for her exciting life ahead with a volleyball scholarship. The binging started immediately upon saying good bye to her. As I drove away, leaving her at the university, I couldn't wait to stop at the next gas station to get a huge supply of stuff to eat for the nine hour drive home. Fear, anxiety, and loneliness overwhelmed me and all I wanted to do was eat. When I got back home too stuffed to feel, I curled up in a fetal position, alone in my daughter's cold empty bed with my metaphorical soother and security blanket (bread and cheese), and there I silently grieved the loss of my last baby to adulthood.

Don't get me wrong, I did NOT want her to stay in Creston and vegetate or marry or work at the local burger joint for the rest of her life. I was happy she was getting on with her life. I just didn't know what this meant for me and what my life would mean now. It's a frightening thing to realize the speed of time and the short span that children are actually children. In my binging grief I chose to focus on everything I had ever done wrong as a parent, plunging myself into a dark place of regret that I tried to blow off with food.

August 30, 2010

Yesterday I left Alicia in Langley to start her university volleyball career. I left her at Trinity Western University around noon then grandma and I drove home. I ate two chocolate bars, a bag of chips, a bunch of cherries, fried chicken, and corn dogs. Ugh. I feel kind of shell-shocked that my parenting days are done. It seems impossible that so many years have passed and my children have grown up.

August 31, 2010

I am hoping I can get my appetite problems under control again and get back into the size ten suit I bought for Joan's wedding last fall. It would be nice to fit it again by the end of the year or sooner. I am focusing on paying attention to hunger signals and full signals so I don't over eat. I am also paying attention to filling my spiritual and emotional needs with spiritual and emotional rewards rather than with food. I feel like my life is beginning again now as I launch myself as a divorced single woman with an empty nest. I feel optimistic and hopeful for a bright future

September 18, 2010

Tonight I am thinking about my trip to San Diego this fall. I have ten weeks before I go and I would like to lose twenty pounds by then. I'm going to start the Tone it Up video again on Monday and do it three times a week besides my walking daily and eating less. I know how to do it and would like to get this past year's gain off again. I would like to fit back into my brown suit before the end of the year. I'm not sure why except that I just feel better without the extra midriff rolls.

# Dream eater

In September I received another blow to my grandiose future plans in the form of a rejection letter from the Mormon Tabernacle Choir. After a food bender and a cry and a prayer I made peace with this blow and put myself out there to God to plan my life one day at a time. It was a time to reflect once again and examine the direction of my life, which apparently remained settled in Creston. No house sale; no dream job; no choir; no children; no diet; no weight loss; just thighs and lost dreams.

To get out of the fat pity party I found myself in I turned again to the twelve-step program for healing.

October 1, 2010 Friday 7:30 a.m.

I am getting myself once again going on the twelve-step program of addiction recovery. Today I'm reading step one on honesty in the LDS addiction manual. I am listing the things that are important to me:

1. Health is very important to me so I am perplexed at why I allow myself to fall into the trap of sugar and overeating so much
2. Spirituality is very important to me. Once again the mystery is why I continue to withdraw from the Spirit by plunging into sugar hell. It's like the

natural woman takes over and I indiscriminately, almost without choice, eat and eat and eat, all the time knowing that what I am doing is damaging my body and spirit.
3. Peace is very important to me. I like to feel the peace that emotional balance brings and when I overindulge and get into food binging that peace leaves and I am left feeling anxious, self-loathing, doubtful, and fearful
4. Hope is important to me. Once again when I eat excessively I become pessimistic and miserable, craving the joys of optimism.
5. Sleep is very important to me. I know how essential sleep is to all of the above and yet when I am overeating my sleep is disturbed. I frequently overeat in the evening and totally destroy my sleep
6. Peaceful relationships. When I am feeling turmoil within myself brought on by my food frenzies, my relationships with others suffer. I feel myself becoming negative, pessimistic, sarcastic, judgemental, and basically just miserable.
7. Looking good and feeling good in my clothes is important to me. When I am overeating, I start gaining and I gain and gain and gain and soon my clothes are too tight or don't fit at all and I am left wearing the same things over and over and over again. I feel self-conscious about my bulges. Ugh.

So if all these things that are important to me are diminished when I start binging, then why do I repeatedly get into this same trap again? Why am I once again twenty pounds more than I was a year ago? This is so insane. I can't believe that I am repeating it so many times. I am going to be 55 next week and I have been living this nightmare food cycle since I was fifteen years old when I went on my first weight loss diet. Silly isn't it? Why can't an intelligent woman like me get a grip on this?

Here's another mystery in my sick brain. I know intellectually that I will feel much happier, calmer, and optimistic if I don't indulge, and yet I feel so anxious thinking that I can't indulge. This is totally ridiculous. It doesn't make any sense. I am doing those very things that undermine my hope of peace and joy and love. Food never was happiness.

What I risk by continuing in my addiction is peace, love, joy, self-esteem, the power of God, hope, development of my talents, positive relationships, my health in all domains, and sleep. There really is a lot at stake if I continue on the path of food addiction. I will not. I cannot reach my God-given potential if I continue this path of food addiction. I know that. I know that in the inner most depths of my soul, so why is the pull of food so powerful? What exactly is so wonderful about sugar, and bread, and cookies, and ... what, what, what?

So the program recommends letting go of pride. Pride distorts the truth about things as they really are. I have felt this many times. Even lately I have tried talking myself into believing that my appearance isn't important or that I can be happy no matter what my weight, or I want to be free to eat whatever I want. Things as they really are would suggest that sugar and its excess eating simply make me feel like crap. I get depressed, insomniac, sarcastic, fearful, and fat when I indulge in the 'freedom' of excess. It is not freedom—it's fear, prison, bondage, misery, and everything else that goes with the loss of the Spirit in my life.

# The horn and hell of plenty

For the Thanksgiving weekend I went to Anacortes to visit my sister. My daughter met me there and we had a fabulously fat weekend together. The power of the food was no match for my abstinence commitment.

<u>October 12, 2010</u>

My sister is a wonderful cook and prepared an amazing feast of turkey, ham, numerous vegetable and potato dishes, and four dessert choices. I ate way too much.

On the trip home from that weekend feast I had a car crash with a moose, hitting it dead-on going about a hundred kilometres per hour. My life flashed before my eyes and all I saw was diets and thighs and scales. At the point of impact I thought about the carrot cake and pies I had brought home with me and hoped they would be okay. They were, and so was I and so was my mom. Alas, my SUV died and that catapulted me into more binging.

<u>Sunday, October 17, 2010</u>

I am still shell shocked about the fact that my children have all grown up. Was I in a fog for 25 years not realizing this was happening, or was I just eating my way through the decades, not knowing that so many years had passed? Food is and has been the constant in my life. It doesn't grow up and leave me. I eat it fast then quickly replace it. Weight loss seems to be a similar story: lose, gain, lose, gain, and lose gain. Every time I am certain that I have finally ended the battle, a new battalion of cellulite rises from the ashes and challenges me to battle one more time. I have even spent some years proclaiming that the fat war was over and the fat won but I can't even stick with that. Here it comes back again and I remind myself that I am still learning.

The hopeful goals set in September were just a bad fat memory as the months ticked away with me filling my time and thighs with food.

November 1, 2010

I am wondering if there is a correlation between excess weight and an excess of possessions. I gave away my living room furniture today because I don't need so much furniture for myself. It's time to pare down possessions and pare down cellulite. I wonder if getting rid of excess possessions will naturally stop excess food consumption and excess weight. I am trying to downsize in more ways than one.

November 8, 2010

I'm not sure why I am so unmotivated to look after my weight. Maybe I'm just plain worn out with worrying about it and never being thin enough, and dieting and dieting and dieting. I just want to be free from the whole scene of dieting and deprivation. I just want to be free of the obsession so I am just trying to exercise more and eat what I want. For the most part I eat very nutritiously.

# More goals gobbled all to fat hell

My trip to San Diego came and went with me having no clothes that fit. Rather than losing those twenty pounds I vowed to lose in the past ten weeks, I had actually gained several. Because I refused to stand on the scale I really don't know what I weighed. I only know that I was fat again; fatter than I had been in a few years. I tried to convince myself that I was a size fourteen but that really was a lie along with all the other lies I was telling myself such as it doesn't matter what size I am, I can be happy.

December 8, 2010

Joan gave me a book on eating clean so I am pondering my fitness and health once again. Joan was an inspiration to me. She and her husband eat well and are very health conscious. I felt a desire to revisit my healthy food practices and get out of my lethargic fat slump. I know that I don't like being stuffed in my clothes. I bought some new clothes to appropriately fit my expanded size which is now fourteen. I need some decent clothes to wear through the winter while I get my body to its right size again. My revolving door of weight issues revolves once again. Let me live it one day at a time and eat for health and vitality and happiness. I remind myself again that sugar never was happiness.

<u>December 10, 2010</u>

It's December 10, 2010 and I am sitting in front of my TV having just polished off a large bowl of ice-cream with raspberries and ground flax seed. I added the raspberries and ground flax seed to assuage some of my guilt for overindulging once again.

I am 55 years old and I have been dieting for about forty years. Frankly I'm exhausted with it, especially considering that here I am fat again. Not only am I exhausted, I am downright mad. No, mad is not a strong enough word for how I feel. I need more syllables, like enraged, infuriated, incensed, embarrassed, ashamed, disgusted, and so much more.

Here I am once again fat. I don't mean grossly obese, but certainly overweight—size fourteen skirts recently purchased for my 5'4" frame. That's probably a bit of a lie because I think I'm really closer to 5'3' than 5'4".

Those skirts were actually very snug and one of them was size sixteen. How deceitful I am! There I was again skirting around the truth and all the time filling my face and butt and thighs.

# Weigh up

December 16, 2010 3:30 a.m.

I have heard it said that the more things change, the more they stay the same. I seem to be closing out this year the same way I closed out last year—overfed, overweight, and overwhelmed with the problem of compulsive eating.

I am 55 years old now and still suffering from problems I identified decades ago. Here I am again, lying awake suffering from excess food. My body can't sleep. It's working so hard to digest and sort out the massive amount of fat-laden, sugar- laden and chemical-laden food that I ate yesterday and last night. I went to a Beam Road potluck Christmas party last night. It was nice to connect and chat with neighbors. I was already stuffed when I got there from the ongoing food available at work and then nuts and cookies at home, then I continued to eat the evening away. Ugh! My poor body is just so over burdened with digestion duties that it's bloating, and gurgling, and flatulating, and suffering. My poor pancreas must be screaming from overuse. I don't know why I inflict such misery on myself.

I feel gross. I am now wearing size fourteen (more like sixteen, but stuffed into fourteen) clothes again. Why can't I figure this out?

I feel shame about my eating problem. I feel embarrassed and sloppy and stupid that I can't seem to stay one size. I'm not sure what this means. Maybe after all these years, I still don't get it, whatever **it** is. Maybe I don't know who I am yet so I just keep trying out different sizes to see which one fits. Maybe I still haven't got it. I feel lazy, stupid, unlovable, sluggish, shameful, and disgusted, like this eating problem is a deep dark secret that I don't want anyone to know about. Yet it's certainly not something that I can hide. It just oozes out again and soon I have multiple chins, thighs, and belly. Even my wrists look fatter today than they did yesterday. Ugh! Alas, I continue to suffer from the effects of the fridge.

Maybe I really don't know what I want. Maybe that's why I can't seem to get it. Don't I want to be fit and lean and healthy? Maybe I'm a liar and a fraud. I keep saying I want this, but maybe I just don't care. I seem to have lost the desire somewhere, but in quiet reflective moments I get it back for a while.

What I would hope for in 2011: So this year, I think I will focus on conquering one thing only—my food problem. 2011 will be my first full year of being alone without the responsibility of children at home. I am going to focus on self-improvement and conquering my food demons. I am drafting a plan for the year. I believe a permanent work position would work well for keeping a steady routine. That would greatly help with eating and exercising.

I would like to take part in some of the fitness programs in the community like yoga, clogging, and water aerobics (if I dare get into a bathing suit). I would like these alternate activities to get out of the house, away from food, and move—something in addition to walking or to replace it on icky winter days.

I need to take care of myself. I am at a point in life where I could seriously damage my physical health if I don't conquer my food demons. So I hope in 2011 to beat my food addiction, to be the size God meant for me to be, to be lean, energetic, and fit. I have a plan: in addition to taking the above fitness programs, I am going to follow *eat clean*. I am going to face the scale on New Year's Day and have Alicia take a picture of me in form fitting clothes. I am going to face the numbers.

# Another year, another diet

I did face the scale and the measurements. Once again I planned another super strict program to beat the weight.

<u>December 21, 2010</u>

Today I have done a trial run of the whole oatmeal breakfast as advised in the *eat clean* diet. I am reminded of mom's voice expounding the benefits of oatmeal porridge. It was basically our standard breakfast fare growing up. The pot of mush. I used to gag it down, promising to myself that when I got old enough to choose, I would never eat oatmeal porridge again. Vain promise. Who'd have thought mom was right all those years? "It sticks to your ribs," she used to promise in her attempt to convert us. Of course we really had no other options. It was eat the oatmeal or starve. Today for the first time since those childhood years I ate a bowl of oatmeal porridge with ground flaxseed, blueberries, and raspberries. No sugar but some cinnamon. I must admit that it wasn't my dream breakfast but I am willing to do whatever it takes for total health once again. I am ready to submit to changes in myself and my lifestyle to have total health. I am doing what is good for me and makes me feel good.

My body is so overloaded right now that I would like to go to some asylum to get away from the excess around me at work, at home, everywhere.

December 27, 2010

It is now time to face the year 2011 and get prepared for some major changes in myself. To prepare for the chalean extreme program I did the fitness tests with Alicia's help and Joan watching on Skype. Then while wearing nothing but a sports bra and Gordon's jock shorts I had Alicia take several shots of me in different poses. Yikes! I had to face the fat and acknowledge to myself that I am fat. It's hard to deny when it's there in a picture easy to see. I am preparing for the year and doing the work.

I swore off sugar once again and set out on another quest for that magic kingdom of eternal slender.

# The diet less travelled

Again I ask, how many flipping day ones can a person have in a lifetime? I guess as many as I want to have and as many as it takes. In fact every day is a new day and holds the potential to be day one. As the saying goes, today is the first day of the rest of my life, so yesterday must have been the last day of whatever that life or diet was.

December 29, 2010

I am taking the road less travelled by choosing to start my NY resolutions today rather than wait until New Year's Day. Three days before NY day to start my resolution to take care of my body once again. I'm not sure why I am starting three days earlier than tradition dictates. But maybe there is something magical about the number three.

I have fought this food addiction now for four decades and it has tormented me, controlled places I have gone, and given me much shame. I am obviously not a balanced person having swung from one extreme to the other for so many decades. I am trying now to be moderate and I know that as long as sugar is in my life I cannot be moderate. It simply has to go. Some people don't have this problem and that is okay. I do and I cannot pretend that I am okay eating whatever and whenever I want because that will get me into trouble. I have tried that strategy and I inevitably end up eating excessively and starting a cycle of binging, self-loathing, poor esteem, deteriorating behavior, and increasing sarcasm. Some people seem to function well with excess weight and they seem to be okay with that. I am not. I hate being fat and no matter what I wear, I don't like being fat.

I'm tired of feeling so desperate to be thin and wanting to hide myself when I'm not.

December 31, 2010

It is now the last day for 2010 and I have faced the numbers on the scale and wondering how I got here again—185 pounds on my 5'4' frame. It is the story of my life from one diet to the next and back again. It seems appropriate to tell my life in sizes, a sugar opera of struggles.

Each day of abstinence from compulsive eating with adherence to clean eating is a huge victory for me. It's like that straight and narrow path that leads to freedom from obsessive compulsive eating. Heaven is freedom to choose. Hell is bondage, bondage to substances, illusions, fears, whatever they may be. The straight and narrow path leads to being straight and narrow—literally. I don't want to be crooked and thick with bulges and cellulite and saddlebags and bat wing arms and belly rolls. I want to be straight and narrow. I am committed to being free from food addiction; from food and fat and flatulence and flab and all the other *f* words that go with it.

Fat is the new *f* word and fifty five is my time to become the fit and fabulous person that I have always wanted to be and what fate has intended me to be. I am free to be me and not what men want or expect me to be.

I am reading in Alma 42 (*Book of Mormon*) and it just dawned on me that Christ descended into hell so that I would not have to and yet I seem to be taking myself into the hell of addiction on a regular basis. The sacrament prayer reminds me every Sunday that Christ descended into hell so that I don't have to. Yet I take a simple substance like food, abuse it, defile it, and gorge on it until it becomes my personal hell. Wake up Ruth and smell the calories, smell the corruption, and consumption and consumerism that have taken food from its source and purpose and give life to a purpose for excess and exploitation.

## As the cellulite turns

I quietly said goodbye to 2010, the year of many losses, none of them fat, and looked forward with a perfect brightness of diet to what a new year would bring for me or take from me. There's something magic about being three days ahead when the New Year starts.

January 1, 2011

New diets are like new boyfriends [like I would know anything about boyfriends, having had really only one and a half my whole life!]. At first there is this phase of 'they can do no wrong' and everything about them is perfect. Then reality sets in and its day to day life dealing with whatever struggles life brings.

January 2, 2011

I am reading Alma 5 (*Book of Mormon*) which talks about God changing hearts. That is what I am desiring and fasting for. That my heart will be changed and I will no longer desire anything contrary to the will of God.

"Behold, he changed their hearts; yea, he awakened them out of a deep sleep, and they awoke unto God. Behold, they were in the midst of darkness; nevertheless, their souls were illuminated by the light of the everlasting word; yea, they were encircled about by the bands of death, and the chains of hell, and an everlasting destruction did await them."

This is how I feel when I am actively 'using' sugar as a drug of choice to deal with life. I feel like I am encircled about by the bands of death and the chains of hell and there is an impending doom of everlasting fat and misery and depression awaiting me. What a terrible image. When I am out of the midst of sugar darkness I feel like my soul is illuminated by the light of Christ. I feel light in many more ways than just physical weight. I feel like a glow with the light of Christ in my body and spirit. The circle of darkness and despair becomes a circle of light and hope.

# Weigh day weigh day

The first weigh in for 2011 came with great glee.

January 5, 2011 179.3 pounds

Yeah, I lost six pounds. I am so excited. I am so excited. I am feeling hopeful and optimistic and grateful that I did not cave to the crave for something else yesterday. I am grateful that I reasoned with myself to remind myself that sugar never was happiness because just for a brief moment, I felt that rebelliousness, that illusion that I couldn't be happy without sugary treats and eating like a normal person. According to the news, over 60% of Canadians are overweight. Do I want to be like a normal person? Obviously it's normal to be overweight so going with the herd is not the happy road. Taking the food less eaten or eating less is the road less travelled. I read somewhere, sometime in my life reads, that the less you eat the better you feel providing what you eat is of high nutritive value. I am feeling the energy and optimism that sugar free eating gives me.

I am sleeping better again and that makes a huge difference to everything else. I eat better, feel better, act better, speak better, and even breathe better. What more can I say? What was I thinking getting sucked into the illusion that sugar is fun and happiness and love……blah blah blah? It's not glamorous or joy or beauty or security and it won't give me my family back. It only separates me from all the wonderful feelings that I want to have: to feel confident and capable and beautiful and healthy. I claim to value my health and yet have once again allowed sugar to overrule that value, so I must admit that when I am using food so inappropriately I am not valuing my health.

I am grateful that I am not crash dieting or starving. A work colleague talked about her HCG supplement diet of five hundred calories a day. All I could think of was how disappointed she will be because such a plan cannot be maintained and is so unhealthy. I have had my share of semi-starvation diets and I know they only bring about more misery. I want to eat well and eat nutritiously. My body has had well enough of years of ridiculous dieting that only made me miserable and I never did get the results of health and beauty that I wanted.

I feel hopeful that this is the year for me to excel and to shine. My goal is to weigh 135 pounds by June 1st.

There you have it in black and white, another weight goal complete with target date eaten all to hell.

# Weigh day weigh day two

Weigh days are not new to me. I've had many, many such days in my diet-laden history. I have it down to a science, whether weighing in the morning, midday, or evening. I neither eat nor drink a thing until after the blessed weigh in. I make sure my bladder and bowels are empty, my nails are clipped (fingers and toes), eyebrows plucked, nose picked, arms and legs shaved, hair bone dry, minimal clothing (naked if possible, tissue g string if not), no jewelry, and lungs fully deflated. Whatever it takes to get that simple psychological edge tipping from .1 to .2 pounds is well worth the agony of preparation.

<u>January 12, 2011 176.88</u>

I lost another 2.4 pounds this week and am very happy with that because after an eight pound loss I was concerned that I might bounce back up again as I have done in previous dieting plans. But this time I didn't and I still continue to eat a substantial amount of food. I am very relieved and happy and feeling hopeful and optimistic.

I keep reminding myself not to sacrifice what I want most for what I want in the moment. What I want is to be lean, fit, trim, and I am thinking about 135 pounds for my height. What I want is to be the size God intended for me to be – whatever that might be.

Maybe it is less than 135, but for now 135 sounds like a reasonable weight for me according to health charts.

# Shooting up with cookies

At my local church an official church sponsored addiction recovery program launched in January and I was excited to be part of it. I worked hard at cleaning up my past and making amends for things I had done and said. My son (then 21) was home visiting for a few weeks and asked me about the meeting I went out to. When I explained it to him, his question was, "Oh mom, what could you possibly be addicted to?"

After explaining my complex decades-old problem with sugar he then asked, "So when did you last shoot up with a cookie mom?" I laughed hysterically, grateful for my son's wonderful sense of humor about his mother's weaknesses. I took the opportunity to apologize to him (making amends) for some past experiences where I felt remorse over events in his life.

In late January I was in Langley to watch my daughter play volleyball and to send my son off again to his exciting volleyball life back in Ottawa. The empty house syndrome loomed again.

January 23, 2011

Now my house is empty and I have had a moment of mother melancholy at the goodbyes of my children again. I'm not sure why I feel so blue each time they leave or I leave them. I am happy that they are developing their talents and moving forward in life. It is a blessing to see them progress. As I have said before, this is my year to change myself and I continue to work on that.

January 30, 2011

Waiting, enduring, dieting, waiting to lose weight certainly is an exercise in patience. I will work and be patient. Soon the winter will be over and staying the course will have me looking great in the spring and summer and beyond. I hope that this is my last time to battle weight cycling and I hope that I can, with the grace of Christ, stay away from binging and the self-loathing and weight gain that goes with it. I feel good. I feel balanced. I feel hopeful. What a difference eating clean makes in my life. I have hope that I can indeed battle this and get my body back down to a healthy weight. When I was blow-drying my hair this morning I looked at my naked body and the rolls of fat on my midriff while I bent sideways. I can't believe I have gained so much weight again. I can't believe how much I am in denial when I start to eat. What the hell was I thinking? Help me remember not to do that ever again.

I am actively working toward the worthwhile goal of weighing 135 pounds and I am not going to get discouraged when results don't appear instantly and without effort. It is happening one clean meal at a time, one walk at a time, one weight lifted at a time. I am patient and looking forward with a perfect brightness of hope.

February 9, 2011 weight 173.14 pounds

I have lost twelve pounds in six weeks – perfect.

I am most grateful for a wonderful sleep last night. A good sleep seems to be the foundation for a wonderful day. I am most grateful for abstinence from compulsive overeating now for 41 days. What a blessing it is to feel free from the obsession with food. My body, mind, and spirit are all happy this morning.

# Strolling down fat memory lane

February 10, 2011

Yesterday I did my weight workout and got going again on my book—poring over old journals having a laugh or two as well as wondering at my ineptness and awkwardness. During my young single years there is a theme of social ineptness and a certain amount of anxiety associated with being single and not being able to relate to men, yet worrying about being single all my life. Alongside this anxiety is my obsession with weight and dieting and never being the right size and always waiting for that magic time in the future when I would be the right size and then all my problems would disappear.

There's also a mix of religious extremism, and many times I would berate myself for not being perfect. I have many entries in which I obsess about my horrible sin and condemn myself because of my mistakes, none of which had the gravity for such self-loathing. I'm not sure if this is all a throw back to my upbringing but I seemed to think that I was very wicked and I'm not sure why I felt that way. I didn't commit any major sins during this time however I am grateful to have these many journals to reflect on and to include in a book of my struggles with weight.

I seem to have spent a lot of my youth anxiously wanting to get married but feeling lost and rejected most of the time, inept at social interaction, and very awkward. Basically I was a social moron especially when it came to relating to guys. I suppose I still am. Part of that was my insecurities about who I am, what I like, and what I want.

February 20, 2011

My home teachers [church ministers] came over this afternoon. They posed the philosophical question, "What do you think would bring you great joy?" "Well", I responded, "I think that I would be pretty joyful if I could eat anything I want and always be a size six—of course, that's a rather carnal joy, isn't it?" Sad, but true.

I am feeling like I want to eat but I am not hungry. I just want to eat all the left over granola bars in the house. I have eaten three today—two before my walk in hopes that my walk would wear them off and now I have eaten a third with my supper. I am actually feeling full and satisfied so may be able to pass this hump. I haven't eaten to excess or compulsively but I have eaten some sugar which is not included in my eat-clean plan. It must be time for me to remember how I like to feel and look. I have been feeling really good, balanced, happy, and peaceful eating clean and I do not want to ruin that now. I am feeling the muscles in my body that I have been developing these past seven weeks of doing weight work. I want to continue to feel this good and not blow it with silly sugar cravings. I want to be lean and healthy and happy.

# Weight expectations

<u>February 25, 2011</u>

I wonder what I expect to gain from being slim. It seems that I have previously thought that all my personal problems could be solved by being slim. Perhaps solving my personal problems first would result in being slim. I have always tried to work from the outside in, believing that if I fixed my outside appearance I would magically have everything else fixed. So what do I expect from being slim? Why is it so important to me that I have been tormented for over forty years with this quest for thinness? I have skipped going to social functions such as my friend's weddings because I did not want to be seen fat. I have avoided many things based on my size at the time. I have let my size dictate my life for many years. I have neglected buying clothes and gone years with just minimal clothing always looking ahead to that magic day when I would buy clothes in the magical size I wanted to be. I would just buy ugly cheap clothes to carry me until that magical time I could be thin and deserve nice clothes. I suppose it has saved me some money on clothing except that whenever I did get down to a comfortable weight I would buy clothing which then sat for years after I quickly gained weight again. I just want to be free from the obsession and have a balanced healthy life.

In early March I travelled to Quebec City to watch my daughter play university volleyball in the nationals for university teams. Thankfully I was able to maintain moderate eating during the trip. From an airport in Toronto enroute home, this next weight reflection occurs.

March 8, 2011

Sometimes I am still tempted to beat myself up when I look at my thighs and belly and see how much I have gained once again but I am learning that beating myself up makes things only worse. I am learning to love and be patient with myself, the same way that I love and show patience for my children. I am okay and I can change one day at a time, one meal at a time, one pound at a time, and one workout at a time. Here I am in my third month now of eating clean and doing weight work. I can celebrate my progress—not perfection. Progress is awesome. Perfection is not realistic in this life.

March 8, 2011

At the Toronto airport I bought *A Course in Weight Loss* by Marianne Williamson. I had heard about the book previously so was happy to see it there. I started reading it on the plane trip, more food for thought on my weight and food and fear issues.

March 9, 2011

Be it ever so cluttered, there's no place like home.

I was annoyed when I stepped on the scale and it was up. Ugh! I feel like I didn't eat much this past week; however it is just a number. Life will go on.

I am working on lesson one in *A Course in Weight Loss*. It is humbling to face my fears, anger, sadness, and to work through them. I hope that I can let go of my emotional issues, love myself, and move forward with a lean and fit body. Love is the cure. I am learning that when I overeat it is a sign of self-hatred and I believe that. To love me is to eat well what I need and take care of my body. I cannot change the past. I can only acknowledge it, learn from it, and move on.

# Hate mail

While doing thought exercises for the book, *A Course in Weight Loss*, I wrote the following letter to my fat self.

March 9, 2011

Dear fat freckled one,

I am writing this letter as required by my course in weight loss. I pity you because I have never liked you. I have always wanted to be thin and you have been the thorn in my flesh that has kept this dream at bay.

I blame you for my poor self-esteem and for my poor behaviors throughout my life. If it wasn't for you, I would not have been rejected by men. When I was in high school, a boy would not have insulted me in front of other guys by saying, 'How sweet it isn't' when I walked by. I felt very humiliated that day, especially because there was a guy there that I had a crush on and I heard all their laughing as I walked by.

I realize that you have been sad and hurt but I really don't like you. I have wanted to be thin all my life as far back as early teens when I thought that without you I could have had a happy teen life and a happy young adult life and I would not have been rejected by the guy I thought was the perfect man. I would also not have been rejected after years of marriage by the one man that actually showed romantic interest in me.

If it wasn't for you I would probably have been popular and happy and everything else that I wanted to be. I would probably also have been more charming and dressed better and even been a decent homemaker.

As it is I feel that you have ruined my life thus far. I feel sorry for you and I realize that you need love just like anyone else. You really embarrassed me when you stole that pizza and coke at work. What were you thinking?

I forgive you for your struggles and I want you to be happy. Please accept my apologies for disliking you. I want you to be happy and feel loved. We all need to feel loved, although I have been afraid of you and your monstrous appetite. I have been afraid that you would never stop eating until you were several hundred pounds and sick and depressed.

I have been scared of your power in my life and always worked hard to keep you under control and to hide you so people did not know about you. I have been ashamed of you. I feel guilty about disliking you but that's the way it is and sometimes I have been so angry that you keep coming back no matter how hard I work to get rid of you.

Why do you keep coming back if I hate you so much? Why don't you stay away when I have dieted and exercised you away? How do you keep coming back so many times over and over and over again? I even left you once in a foreign country—all the way to Asia without a passport and you still came back and found me. Then I ditched you in Hawaii years later and you came back so fast I couldn't remember living without you. Why, why, why won't you stay away when I get rid of you? How can you be so powerful over me as to ruin so much of my esteem? I want to like myself but I find it hard to do when I see your thighs and belly rolls and double chins ruining my pictures.

Just when I get new clothes to fit my slim self, you turn up again and ruin my wardrobe. I just don't get it. Why won't you stay away when I don't want you?

I hate to be rude—well, maybe I like to be rude. Butt out of my life and let me live slim.

Yet I realize that you have deep feelings of wanting to be seen and heard. I think that you have felt invisible and ignored much of your life and I am sorry for you. I believe that you have the right to be heard and seen and loved.

I have missed social engagements because of you. I didn't want to be seen when I was fat. I skipped a friend's wedding reception in Creston because of you and every year that I was fat I refused to go out and I refused to dress well and I refused to wear makeup and live. I was always waiting to get rid of you before I could really live and here I am, still waiting to get rid of you. I'm still waiting for that magical day when I will be thin and then I will start to live. It seems that I have spent my whole life looking forward to being thin and had only brief glimpses of this then you would come back with a vengeance and ruin my thinness.

Although I must thank you for continuing to work out, walk, hike, bike, climb the Grand Canyon, work, and put up with my food and mood swings. Thank you for being there for me through it all no matter what I did to you. I appreciate your tenacity and health.

Signed,

The thin wannabe

# PS I love me

Another exercise for the course in weight loss was to write a response from my fat self to the thin self I wanted to be. The fat freckled one writes back.

March 19, 2011

Dear Thin Wannabe,

I have worked hard for you to digest and assimilate all that food you shoved into me. I am not responsible for your poor eating choices and binges and hate. I have basically been your garbage dump when you hated yourself and ate and ate and ate and ate. I am here because you have created me and I don't like to be hated by the very one who created me. Lighten up with your hate and I will lighten up period.

Let me live and be happy and feed me the whole foods of the earth and I will respond with the exact body you want. I do not ask or pine to be fat. I am at your mercy and the mercy of your binging when you're upset with yourself. Don't hate me or yourself. There is love for both of us and it is love that will heal us.

How do you think I feel supporting and carrying and digesting for you all these years and hated just the same? I conceived, carried, nurtured, and grew beautiful children for you and then they fed at my ample breast for the first years of their lives. I provided that nourishment for them. I have continually carried you on your monster walks and hikes at all sizes and have continued to support you.

I carried you to the depths of the Grand Canyon and back up again—remember your thin self was not there. It was I who did that and I continue to carry your load and walk and cycle and weight lift you all over. How can you hate someone who does that for you?

And all those guys who rejected you or didn't notice you? Screw 'em. They don't deserve you. What a marvelous person they missed when they rejected you and now you are going to show them. They failed to see the magnificent beautiful person you are. Now expose that beautiful person for the one God intended for you. It's not over. It's your time to shine for all to see and your beauty, grace, charm, and talent will absolutely stun them. 'Huh!?' they'll say, 'Where did she come from? I did not see that coming!' You go girl—it's your time to shine. It's your turn.

Go with God, the One who loves you and knows you, and all will be well.

In the deepest sincerity of my heart,

Signed,

Fat Freckled Little Girl—the plain one, the easy keeper, the good doer, the husky one.

P.S. Don't think I don't remember all those labels over the years from visitors and relatives and don't think I didn't know that someday I would shock them all with my beauty, wit, charm, grace, and talent. Here goes.

# And Ruth said

March 18, 2011

I have spent sometime this morning reviewing my journal and continuing obsession with food. Today I wake feeling the peace of abstinence in my life. It is a good feeling to be free from the effects of compulsive eating and to know I have honored rather than desecrated my body with food. It's like I wake up to a genuinely new day rather than waking up still packing the negative effects of yesterday with me. What a blessing it is not to pack yesterday's leftovers into today and have to start this day already burdened and behind from the food baggage of yesterday. No wonder I feel so light and free on mornings when I wake up free of yesterday's excess.

It's hard to live one day at a time when you're packing several days' worth of food along on your body and, I might add, on my mind as well. I know from experience that food does not just weigh heavily on the body but also on the mind and spirit. This emotional and spiritual cellulite is even more troubling than the physical bulges accumulating on the hips, thighs, belly, arms, toes etc. Even though these physical unsightly bulges are the most evident, it is the bulges accumulating in my heart and soul, robbing me of the peace of God, that are infinitely more distressing and destructive. The humiliating turmoil I feel on the inside is far more debilitating than what others may see on my outside.

I bought some dinner plates with scriptures on them. How cool is that? Perhaps if I have a scripture on the very plate I am eating off of I will be strengthened in my battle against compulsive overeating. I feel strengthened just thinking about it. The purchase of the plates is a suggestion from a *Course in Weight Loss*. I am to purchase a beautiful dinner plate just for me to start my love affair with food.

Initially I may have thought that my weight issues meant a need to find me; now I know that I need to find God. He's not lost, I am, and the closer I get to Him the closer I get to me. He is my creator and knows me – all of me—the fat, the thin, the in between. The more I know God, the more I know myself as created in His image. As I fill my cells with His divine light I lose my desire to fill them with excess food. I am grateful for another day of abstinence from compulsive overeating.

# Hook line and sugar

March 23, 2011

The best preparation for a good day is a previous good day, defined for me as one free from compulsive eating. That was yesterday for me. I lived and ate free with clean food.

This is my self-designated weigh in day and I am disappointed that the number on the scale has gone up from last week. This is when the weigh day weighs heavily on my mind. How can I be up on the scale when I feel light and fit and sure that I am leaner than last week? This is where I have to come up with some acceptable explanation so as not to give up in despair and say it's not worth it. That stinky thinking will take me straight into a food binge which will further spiral me into the abyss of food hell and misery that I have so struggled with all my life. So let me bask in feeling fit and lean even though the scale does not support my feeling. Perhaps my muscles are developing and weighing more than the fat I am losing. I may be leaner and smaller while the numbers on the scale don't show it. That's my soul soothing story and I'm sticking to it. Somewhere, sometime, the numbers will again go down and my mood will again go up. Just for today I am not going to let this mood-weight inverse relationship ruin my months of abstinence and peace. No more will the scale dictate my mood and motivation for the day. Awake my soul, no longer droop in sugar. Today I celebrate feeling hope, peace, and joy.

I just saw a McDonald's ad for their new filet of fish sandwich. It boasts, 'Just one bite and you'll fall for it hook line and sinker.' Now if that isn't an addiction, I don't know what is. I can bet that it's not the fish that hooks, lines, and sinks. I don't really like that image for food. Hooking me and sinking me has fat addiction written all over it. I don't want to be hooked, lined, or sunk. I want food that liberates, lightens, and lifts rather than sinks me. Sucks to be McDonald's. Just goes to show you they know their food is addictive. Who wants to be hooked and lured into the bondage of fat and salt and grease and plugged arteries and bowels?

March 27, 2011

I like this verse in Romans 6:6

*Knowing this, that our old man is crucified with him, that the body of sin might be destroyed, that henceforth we should not serve sin.*

It seems to me that this verse is telling me that my old self, the obsessive compulsive eater, was crucified with Christ, but I keep dragging her up and feeding her and resuscitating her and hauling her around in my attitude and mind and emotion. Why am I continuing to drag around the old negativity that Christ died to deliver and redeem? Sure doesn't make any sense to me. I also remind myself that He did this for others too, so why should I bring up their old sins and relish in them and share them and keep them alive? That which is gone is gone. Let it die.

Sometimes I think that I should not bother God with my seemingly insignificant problem of food addiction citing major world disasters as more important to Him. In this I am limiting His power as if He has to choose one problem or person over another to help. His power is sufficient for every need to be satisfied in all the world, so when I am accessing His power to overcome food addiction I am not taking that power away from others who also need it. He is all powerful for all the world. My concerns are just as valid as any other.

# The fat tormentors

April 11, 2011

I am reading the Sunday school lesson on who is my neighbor and about forgiving others. I am impressed with the phrase in Matthew 18 being delivered to the tormentors when we don't forgive others, for Christ forgives us. I do not want to be delivered to the tormentors so I forgive all things. Today I will ponder this thought and remember it when I am tempted to feel grudging thoughts. Being delivered to the tormentors does not sound pleasant. It sounds akin to being plunged again into food hell, with my head buried in a bag of chips while my hands cling to chocolates and pizza and cookies and so forth while my belly churns and torment settles in. Please do not deliver me to the tormentors.

Torment for me would certainly be food hell, fat hell, flatulence hell, fear hell.

I got a rejection letter from a magazine for the Christmas article I submitted. Darn! I felt down for a while and might have given in to eat something, but I resisted the temptation. I wouldn't want to blow abstinence and recovery over a magazine rejection.

I am struggling tonight with a desire to eat beyond the bounds of my physical needs. I am not sure why.

May 4, 2011

Today my weight is 161.9 pounds, so I have now lost 23 pounds in eighteen weeks. Slow and steady. Slow and steady. I wore my size ten denim capris today and they were not too tight. Doing weights has certainly trimmed me down and I am grateful for that. It feels good. One day at a time.

May 11, 2011 Wt. 160.6 pounds

Look at that. I have lost almost 25 pounds since January 1st and I have done it with a comfortable eating plan. I had a few small sugar splurges but have resisted mostly with the grace of God through the addiction recovery program. Thank thee Lord for this victory thus far.

I never arrive. There's no such thing as arriving. It's all a continuum to eternity.

May 18, 2011

My weight is up this week. I felt it coming. Ugh. I've been compromising what I eat, letting in too much sugar and salt and then expecting to work it off. It does not work. I cannot out train bad eating habits. I must refocus. I've also had too much aspartame and diet pop. It all contributes to increased eating and cravings. Turn it around now, turn it around now. I am reminded of a friend saying, 'You don't have to ride all the way to the dump before you get off the garbage truck.'

1:00 p.m. I am still struggling to keep from eating. There was a mistake made on my pay check so the first thing I want to do is eat. What exactly am I feeling? Am I feeling persecuted? Am I feeling scared? Am I feeling hopeless? What exactly am I feeling at this moment? For some reason I want to eat. I am feeling a bit of anxiety about the realtor coming and signing an agreement. I am feeling scared of being taken advantage of. I have never been very good at advocating for myself. I feel selfish and embarrassed if I advocate for myself. I am going to go outside now and water my plants and maybe the sun and fresh air will help ease the urge to eat.

8:30 p.m. I think it did help, going out for fresh air.

The pull of food has lessened a bit and I have not eaten since supper which was a balanced moderate meal.

I panicked a bit about some old thinking that tried to creep in to my head, that old thinking that I can eat a bit of sugar; I can eat what I want. I can nibble a bit here and there and it won't matter. It does matter and I need to remind myself that it does matter. The numbers on the scale today show that it does matter.

# Ruth, where art thou?

May 29, 2011

There was lots of food around at work. While I didn't get into the sweets, I did eat more cheese and buns than needed at supper. I was feeling bad about myself over a mistake I made at work. It seems to be a pattern: whenever I feel bad about myself I react with self-destruction. Excess food is self-destruction. It's very uncomfortable to dislike myself. I don't like feeling stupid and berating myself. I need to simply accept that I make mistakes and hope to learn from them. I need to let it go and accept today. I am not living yesterday. Now I am living today.

May 30, 2011

(2 Nephi 27:3 *Book of Mormon*). I am likening this scripture unto me. I have eaten many times but my soul is empty. I have attempted to fill my soul with physical food and that cannot be done. My soul needs spiritual food, which I am seeking now. My soul has an appetite different from my body and I have confused these two for most of my life that I can recall. I have been drunken but not with wine. I have been drunken with food. I have staggered but not with strong drink; I have staggered with excess food. I have closed my

eyes to the truth of who I am and my Source for peace. Simultaneously I have opened wide my mouth and stuffed myself with food—hiding who I am from myself and from others. I have rejected the Creator by rejecting myself.

I would rather suffer abstinence and know God than to enjoy the pleasures of sugar for a season. The pleasure of sugar is not worth the pain.

By faith the walls of my pride and fat will come tumbling down and I will see through a glass clearly. I will see who I really am: the offspring of God created in His image and not my own. I belong to God. All that I am and all that I have belong to God. Through faith my food addiction will be subdued and my lion mouth shall be stopped. Out of my weakness I will be made strong, turning to flight from the armies of sugar. I have been tempted and spiritually slain by sugar, wandering about in multiple sizes of temporary clothing, turning aside from the beauty of spiritual raiment that has been promised and being spiritually destitute, afflicted, and tormented. I have wandered in worldly diets, spiritual deserts, and hidden myself in dark caves of earthly excess. My soul has cried out in drought and I have stuffed it with sugar and cruelly silenced it rather than allowed it to soar on spiritual nourishment.

(2 Nephi 27: 27 *Book of Mormon*). I have sought deep to hide myself from God and who I am meant to be. I have eaten myself into a dark hole, the depths from which only God can redeem me. I have hidden and isolated myself in my addiction, eating when no one was looking, and sought to keep myself hidden with

my shameful habit of stuffing myself to the point of nausea and vomiting then being filled only with shame. The problem is that this addiction does not hide for it shows so blatantly in the size of my thighs and my chin and my butt and my belly and all things of a bodily nature. It also shows in my countenance that I am miserable in my addiction. What I have done in the darkness of isolated eating shows in all aspects of my physical world. Indeed, it cannot be hid for long.

June 1, 2011

My precious Alicia is nineteen years old today. How can nineteen years go by so fast when dieting for a week seems an eternity?

# Cerebral cleansing

June 12, 2011 7:00 a.m.

I just read this scripture: Psalm 119:28 *My soul melteth for heaviness: strengthen thou me according unto thy word.*

I have had many days, weeks, months, even years of melting my soul with heaviness. More aptly put, eating heaviness to my soul through excess and pretend food.

While pondering my many spurts at weight loss via cleansing regimes (i.e. elderberry cleanse, fruit fasting, water fasting, cabbage soup cleanses etc.) it dawned on me that what I needed to cleanse was my mind and then my body would follow suit. It's not so much the colon that needs cleansing as it is my cognition. Cognition cleansing is my new buzz phrase, or cerebral cleansing. Maybe that sounds more like it.

June 14, 2011

Yeah, I am 159.94 pounds this morning. I have finally cracked into the 150s. I am so excited, I am so excited. I feel ripped and healthy and light.

June 20, 2011

I just listened to a news clip about obesity in Canada. Most people they say under-report their weight. DUH! Of course we do, we don't want to be that fat.

July 6, 2011

I am now down to 158 pounds—that is a 27 pound loss in 27 weeks. It looks like my overall average loss is a pound a week for some reason. I had hoped as usual that it would be faster. Isn't that what we all dream? Make me twenty pounds less by next week when I have a reunion coming up? Anyway, in hindsight one pound a week does add up and time does fly. I feel content with my manner of eating and do not feel a compulsion to dive into anything fattening or junky or sweet, so I feel very blessed about that. I also continue to get a lot of exercise—most days, at least two hours of biking, walking, weights, or DVD cardio. I am building a lot of muscle and strength. I can almost fit into a sage green suit I have that is size ten so I know that the weight work has made me leaner than I normally would have been at this weight. I usually do not get into that suit until I am below 150 pounds I can see though where I need to get off another twenty pounds of fat and I can do that living the way I am.

# Satisfy my soul in diet

July 25, 2011

Psalm 86: 13 *For great is thy mercy toward me: and thou hast delivered my soul from the lowest hell.*

For me, the lowest hell is total bondage to physical appetite which inevitably becomes a state of anxiety, misery, worry, fear, doubt, and self-hatred. It is the lowest hell for me because when I hate myself I seem to hate everyone else. Bitterness and hatred are a hellish misery go round to be on. Such is the misery of food hell. No food or food product is worth the pain of food hell.

July 27, 2011

Reading in Acts 3 about the lame man healed. He went walking and leaping and praising God. That's how I feel with abstinence and each pound loss. I lost another pound this week and I feel like walking and leaping and praising God. Well I have actually already had a walk this morning, but I am going to leap and praise God with each pound lost.

July 29, 2011

Proverbs 18:21 *Death and life are in the power of the tongue.*

I know this scripture is referring likely to our words and speech, but for me it could also be food, the power of my tongue to eat dead or living foods and subsequently experience life or death.

# The ties that binge and gag

August 5 2011

I had a good day at work then went to the family reunion. I saw relatives that I have not seen for a long time. I confessed to my aunt about taking white bread and eating to excess while staying at her place when I was a child. She just laughed. I told her I had never had white bread before and I could not seem to stop eating it and stuffing myself with it so I snuck bread between meals and ate and ate and ate. She just laughed some more. I guess I was confessing and trying to make restitution.

August 6, 2011

I am grateful that I did not cave into the cookies and squares and white buns at last night's reunion bash. I felt relaxed and enjoyed the people rather than focusing on the food. Now I can awaken feeling light and refreshed and confident that I can maintain abstinence again today by seeking out people and engaging them in meaningful conversations. I am going to relax and enjoy family rather than food. It doesn't have to be all about the food, although the anticipation of the dreaded homemade monster cinnamon buns is somewhere in the back of my brain. Better there than sitting on my thighs. I am going to do my work out first before heading out to the park. I am not going to go for the breakfast, which is waffles, strawberries, cream, and such. I just can't seem to think that would be a good idea for an addict such as myself.

August 7, 2011

Yesterday was another day of reunion food and now I need to analyze the day and how it went and the feelings that went with it. I was holding out well through most of the day. I played a round of bucket golf with my cousin, his wife, and daughter in law. Then I had a moderate lunch when that came around. I avoided the cookies and Rice Krispy squares that were everywhere. I focused on visiting with relatives that I have not seen for years and listened to the updates of their families.

Anyway, my stealing of the white bread from my aunt seemed to be a good joke again for her family and they had a few more laughs about that yesterday.

Things in my food department were going well through mid-afternoon. I sat relaxed enjoying the family auction. After the auction they brought out the cinnamon buns. I avoided those until a friend arrived. We chatted for a while. She is perennially underweight and as she shared some of the family dysfunction in her life, I felt tension. I am not sure what I really felt. She had a cinnamon bun while we visited and before long I was eating one too. The strange thing is that I really didn't enjoy it. I would have enjoyed it more had it been filled with flax seed and whole grain but I ate it anyway. Immediately I wanted another one. I felt more tension at the presence of some cousins on the other side of the family. They were not part of the clan but had stopped to see us. For some reason I felt discomfort with them there. I think that because after the initial hug and how are you, there really is nothing left to chat about and I felt awkward. What do you do then? All these relatives are part of the past really and have vastly different lives than I now have. Anyway, after the initial cinnamon bun I fought my food demons for a while.

Some unpleasant memories associated with the people I saw surfaced and I reminded myself that I am no longer a child and it's okay for me to choose who I want to be with now. Maybe I felt uncomfortable because I was sort of pretending to be happy to see people that really are not part of my life and that I really don't care to see. I don't like having to be in pretend mode. I hugged them, had polite conversations with them, and then wondered how I could politely get away from them. Don't get me wrong: I don't wish them ill or anything. It's just that, beyond the superficial, what do you say?

Patterns of behavior associated with family dysfunction are difficult to break when in the presence of family from the past. I lost my focus with the cinnamon bun and felt the terrible compulsion to eat and eat and eat and eat as though I was that little girl who had no control over her life and had to be what others expected her to be. I reined in these feelings talking constantly to myself that the past is past. I am now who I choose to be. I don't have to be what I think others expect me to be. I can be me. It's okay. No one is going to force me to be something or someone else.

I am also ashamed that I was relieved that some relatives did not come, but I pretended to be disappointed when it was brought up. Being pretentious really annoys me, especially when I am the one being pretentious.

So I feel guilty about not wanting them in my life and I guess I still harbor bitter feelings toward them for the way they treated my children and for their arrogance. I am ashamed of the feelings and think I have overcome them until they surface when the conversation turns to them again. Not sure what to do with this, but I have admitted openly to God these feelings (as if He doesn't know!). I am going to discuss them with a friend this week.

What does all of this have to do with eating? I know that I eat when I am not being authentic or when I feel a threat to my self-concept, which is when I am around people from my past and people I have had difficulty with. Of course, family is right up there because family is who have shared the biggest part of the journey with me—'the ties that bind and gag', as Erma Bombeck says. I might add, the ties that also reflect and resonate and remember and judge. So much of who I am has been my relationship with siblings and I have a lot of them.

Getting back to the cinnamon bun, I almost caved into the crave and the self-loathing, but tried to refocus. I was grateful to leave the conversation with the person where I started the cinnamon bun. Thankfully another relative started to chat with her and I made a polite exit and turned attention elsewhere. It's not that I do not like the person I was chatting with. I do like her and respect her but felt a need to eat when she ate and felt tension in the conversation.

When the talent show started, my sister informed me that she had put us on the program to sing *Sentimental Journey*, so we did this impromptu and it was okay. I relaxed and enjoyed the talent show, always cognisant of the food monster trying to take over my soul and a few cinnamon buns sitting nearby on the table. Damn those people who can take a bite and leave the rest! That is my friend with whom I was talking when the cinnamon bun ended up in my mouth. She is perennially thin and asked for half a cinnamon bun and ate it slowly then left some. This is probably what really irritated me so I ate. How can she do that? I do not understand. Maybe I subconsciously thought that I could eat like that and look like her, although she really is too thin. Anyway, I was well aware of the cinnamon buns nearby and when the talent show was over I found myself reaching and picking at one. I didn't have to sit right by the cinnamon bun but that's where I was. My brother asked who's bun it was, to which I replied, 'I don't know,' but there I was picking at it just like my thin friend, pretending I could do that and not gain weight. He then wanted it, so I grudgingly passed it on to him and bitterly watched him eat the rest of it, partly relieved but more angry that I was not eating it.

Soon after, the supper was ready and I felt a compulsion to eat and eat and eat. I kept reminding myself that it's not about the food. It's about family and connecting and visiting, but the food demons seemed to be louder than the family connectors. There was a veritable war going on in my members—the brain divided bitterly in a dispute over compulsive eating and the stomach screaming both yes and no, while my pancreas screamed no. As I waited in line, pretending to chat and be interested in people, my brain was fighting a battle of epic proportions—the battle over food addiction. As I neared the food, the tension was rising. Would I eat clean or would I cave to the crave, throw calories to the waist, and all out binge? The suspense was killing me silently with a spoon while those around me visited superficially. No one was suspecting the battle that was raging in my soul.

My siblings were serving as I approached the bench, the bar of food addiction where battles are waged, won, and lost in a single spoonful. I took the meatballs, eating one immediately and compulsively while asking for a second helping. I passed on the mashed potatoes, taking a bun instead, some Caesar salad, and a few raw veggies and dip and a small piece of chicken.

I wanted to gorge myself and I wanted to run. Like Joseph who was sold into Egypt by his brothers and fled from the temptation of Potiphar's wife, I wanted to bolt from the temptation of the food. Forget sex and body parts, it's all about the fresh baked buns and butter and huckleberry jam and mashed potatoes.

In an instant a vision of myself fat and waddling and miserable and alone and isolated and self-loathing swept through my dopamine-ridden brain. I tried to calm myself and eat slowly but already I was thinking about that birthday cake I had seen in the kitchen, knowing that it was still to come. I went back to get a second bun with butter and huckleberry jam. I came back to my senses when I realized I did not really enjoy it and I did not get the dopamine rush I was expecting. I stopped and paused and tried to refocus.

Mom sat beside me with cake and ice cream. There were three flavors. I wanted an enormous cone with all three flavors. No, I wanted to take the buckets home and binge freely (no such thing as freedom when I get that way—it's more like binge in bondage) through the night.

Just then Marshall texted me and said he was at the house locked out. I took it as an excuse to leave, which I did. I went home, leaving the cake and ice cream and dopamine there. I sat briefly and visited with him then went to bed. Today is another day to wage the fight against food addiction. Today I can go to church and feel a spiritual boost in my life. Just for today I will practice peace and trust in the power of God to deliver me from the food monster. I am grateful that I did not stay and eat ice cream and cake. I am grateful that I did not continue to eat when I got home last night. I am grateful that today is a new day and I will now go forward, accepting that one day at a time is all I need to live.

7 p.m. I found a cinnamon bun in the garbage and took it out and ate it. It must have been thrown in there by someone last night. It was so good even though it was kind of dried out and taken from the kitchen garbage. It was basically clean garbage and my garbage, as disgusting as it sounds to pull a cinnamon bun out of the garbage and eat it. I had a dopamine rush as soon as I saw it. All that was between me and that eternal gulf of misery and woe called food hell. The tug of war between soul and cellulite continues on.

## August 15, 2011

Here's another great line from Romans 7:18 *For I know that in me (that is, in my flesh,) dwelleth no good thing: for to will is present with me; but how to perform that which is good I find not.*

That no good thing which dwells in me and wants to destroy me is my pride—rearing its ugly heart and head and tongue to destroy my peace with eating. Don't eat; pray to have this wicked compulsion rooted out of my breast and thighs and butt and heart and belly. As the great Lamanite king so aptly speaks in Alma 22, (*Book of Mormon*) I would give up all that I possess to have this affliction gone forever to know that I could be in joyful recovery forever and never again feel the misery of food addiction, grabbing and clinging and foraging desperately and relentlessly for that next sugar fix or bread fix or whatever fix it is that I need to hide myself and my pathetic insecurities.

Pride has literally been weighing heavily on my soul—or thighs and belly and butt. I want to be stripped of pride. I believe that I really do, however perhaps I don't want the pain associated with the stripping.

# Double chins, double minded

August 27, 2011

Silence in writing usually means that I am avoiding the scale or denying or ignoring what has happened. What has happened usually is that I have relapsed to using my drug of choice—food. I had a family barbecue on Thursday. It was a beautiful day. Something about hosting meals that is very anxiety-inducing for me, probably because I don't feel confident with such things.

Even though it was family only, I usually have some anxiety about whether there will be enough food and whether I will burn or otherwise maim the food in some way or that people will not show or too many people will show or that the ones who do show will feel awkward in each other's presence. Then there was Alicia's boyfriend here and I wonder what his assessment of the whole dynamics might be. It's probably just typical family dynamics and such. It turned out okay as far as I can tell. I ate my anxiety away, which is an indicator of my own insecurities. I had some peach pie with frozen yogurt and as I ate all I could think of is how I could sneak some more after everyone left.

I felt the stress of hypocrisy, having expounded the evils of sugar so many times but secretly wanting to eat all that left over peach pie that my sister-in-law brought. I don't even know why I asked her to bring peach pie except that I was romancing the notion of a rendezvous with that pie when everyone left me alone. As it turned out, my sister and I had another piece later when most of the guests had gone. I still wanted more. My sister has never had a weight problem, while I, the fat one, have always struggled, but I'M not bitter! Then my precious baby left at night to drive with her boyfriend to Kelowna. I took my overburdened belly and heart and went to bed.

Predictably I woke up in the early morning hours with my binge headache and broken heart and took some Excedrin. I got up and went for a huge hike with Marshall, hoping to burn off some of that pie while mending my broken heart. Sounds like a bad country western song.

Then I went to work for six pleasant hours. I got home from work, ate the rest of the pie with some sugar free ice-cream (alone again), and went out for a three hours bike ride—again trying to burn off the excess. I realize that I am feeding my extremes with such behavior. Binge exercising trying to balance out binge eating— my life and cellulite hanging in the balance. Now the pie is gone.

August 28, 2011

I am sitting out on my deck enjoying the beautiful evening and temperature after another hot day. I'm not sure why I had a little eating spurt here this evening, likely because of the availability of food. There were leftovers still from my BBQ last week: whole grain flax chips and sugar free ice-cream. I hope this relapse is over as of right now. I still feel kind of lethargic and blah, probably the food hangover.

# By small and simple sugars are great thighs brought to pass

August 31, 2011

I faced the scale this morning after two weeks of avoiding it, knowing that I have not been eating clean. The food compulsions are evidenced in the numbers on the scale. I am up another pound from two weeks ago when I was up a pound from the previous week. It is so frustrating how quickly I can start packing weight back on when my eating changes. In the past two weeks I have continued to get a fair amount of exercise and yet up goes my weight with too much food. Ugh! As soon as I start eating sugar or refined carbs I start expanding no matter how much exercise I get.

Today is as good a day as any to stop this cycle once again. I need this focus today. Today is a crucial day for me. I can nip this binge in the pound rather than wait for it to be ten pounds or twenty pounds or thirty pounds I have to stop it now. I know that I have a lifetime of binges left in me but I don't know if I have another recovery in me. Just for today I will abstain from compulsive eating. Armed with the power of God, I step out into the war on weight.

September 6, 2011

I cannot risk one more fat/sugar offensive against my body.

September 15, 2011

I had a real pity party this morning after a disturbing conversation, in which a person said some rather cruel things about one of my children and their alleged past behavior. I felt that the comments were exaggerated and one sided and cruel, sparking a host of regrets and sadness in my soul. I am very sensitive to attacks on my children, especially by the people in this instance whom I felt were rather arrogant and self-righteous about their own children. The four chambers of my heart have been outside my body since the birth of my four children. I wear my heart out there wherever they go.

I cannot change the past. It is past. It is gone. Please take this bitterness from my soul and thighs and cellulite and belly and whatever other body part it wants to cling to. I feel rather beat up emotionally and it hurts so I will cry instead of eat. I thought this was past and that I could just let it all go but apparently I have not really let it go—I have not arrived. Its times like this that I would like to move away and be far removed from life in Creston. But alas, here I am sitting in an enormous house. Still bitter after all these years. Why is that so? I do not know. I will continue to work out the bitterness with the fat and sugar and everything else that seems to be blocking my spirit from its source of creativity and joy.

It is now near 9:00 p.m. and I have struggled all day with my bitter feelings praying off and on to have them go and trying to fight them. I am grateful that I did not allow my bitterness to compel me to eat the cookies at work. I stayed true to abstinence today.

# Size most certainly DOES matter

September 26, 2011

I tried on my black size eight cord skirt and it fit. I am so excited!

September 27, 2011

I was so excited about fitting into my skirt last night that I could not get to sleep. I kept feeling my body and how good it felt slim and fit. I could feel my lower body muscles and it felt good, but I lost sleep over it. This morning I am reading in Alma 55 (*Book of Mormon*), and this line applies to my food issues. It is pleasant to my taste so I eat the more freely. Should I write that in the past tense? At any rate, when it's really pleasant to my taste I seem to have difficulty stopping.

October 21, 2011

What is it about fall that makes me want to hunker down and gain weight. What is it about the shorter days that trigger a desire for food? It seems that as the light decreases, my appetite increases and I struggle more to keep my cravings at bay. I want to eat and I don't want to eat. I want to eat but I don't want the consequences. In short, I want literally to have my cake and chips and cookies and chocolates and eat them too. I am struggling to battle these desires. Today being a 12-hour work day and now near the end I am wanting to eat. I am going to go home in an hour and I am going to go straight to my lean circuit work out and do that then climb into bed and go to sleep. I have to work again tomorrow so I want to just workout then sleep. I desperately do not want to cave into the food crave again and eat myself fat again before the end of the year.

October 26, 2011

Ephesians 4:14 *no longer carried about by every wind of doctrine.* In my case, no longer carried about by every wind of dieting or sucked into every diet trick and pill and gadget and gogi berry or acai berry or whatever else magic berry that comes along, but balanced and grounded in the wisdom and greatness of God. Every worldly diet does lie in wait to deceive, – only interested in my money and not my weight management or my health. I am no more tossed to and fro by these cunning deceivers sucking me in with all their magical weight loss plans. The only thing that has ever got long term slimness from such plans is my bank account, certainly not my thighs.

# The naked truth

November 3, 2011

I am reading in Mormon chapter nine about judgement day and being brought to see my own nakedness before God. That's a humbling thought. Nothing can be hidden then. No scarves in the right place or slimming lines or colors or any other flaw-hiding device or trick will work. I will be as I am, naked before my Maker and He will see exactly what I have done with His creation. Yikes! I hope I will be found lean and fit and bulge-less or cellulite-less in that great and dreadful day. I wish I could say of my weight that there has been no variableness or shadow of changing but the truth is that my weight and I have been constantly changing up and down and up and down. I am feeling the effects of fall and darkness and too much work and wanting to eat.

Halloween came and went without me eating the treats at work but I have been struggling since having a dinner for mom on Sunday. I ate chocolate cake and apple pie. My sister left her leftover apple pie and ice cream so I ate the rest of that. For the past three days I have eaten some sugar free ice cream and berries each evening and have eaten beyond necessity. I have got to stop this pattern now or I will quickly explode again.

I am most aware that I could gain all my lost weight from the past ten months in the next two months leading up to Christmas. Now is the time to repent and change or I will be fat again. I have another fat binge in me but I don't know if I have another recovery.

# Stop the fatness

November 4, 2011

I feel negative weight habits creeping back into my life and must stop them from destroying my peaceful abstinence. I am eating a bit more sugar then not wanting to weigh in because of fear that weight is up then not wanting to wear pants that just fit for fear they don't anymore. So I weighed this morning and yes, it is up to 155 again, so I have got to stop this upward movement on the scale and get out of the negative rut again. Cut the rut and stop the pattern of behavior before it ends up taking over my life again.

Alicia posted a picture of her and me taken last winter at one of her games. Yikes! I look enormous; my face and neck look so huge. It reminded me why I was eating a bowl of grass for lunch. I definitely do NOT want to look like that ever again! I look horrible, huge. It made me more motivated to keep from putting the weight back on.

November 8, 2011

Reading Ether (*Book of Mormon*) is a bit like reading my life journal. The cycle of pride, prosperity, and wickedness could be likened to my cycles of pride, binging, and dieting. The cycle in both happen so fast that my head and thighs are spinning.

Noah and some of the other Old Testament prophets lived for centuries, so if I lived for centuries would I still be dieting and binging or would I finally conquer, say in about the 400th year of my life?

November 11, 2011

I am reading in Mormon chapter nine and likening the scriptures unto me. I hope in that great day to be loosed from the bands of dieting. The scriptures talk of that great Day of Judgement when she that is filthy shall be filthy still and she that is righteous shall be righteous still and she that is happy shall be happy still and I add she that is fat shall be fat still and she that is lean shall be lean still. I hope I am found lean and without cellulite in that great day. God has not ceased to be a God of miracles and my miracle is a daily reprieve from compulsive overeating.

I have been like a wave of the sea driven by the winds of worldly wisdom and tossed about by every new diet fad that came along. Ever tossed about between feast and famine, never settled in my heart, ever wavering back and forth and up and down and in and out. I have trusted in dead diets.

# More of the cellulite piled higher and deeper

<u>November 16, 2011 152.68 pounds</u>

Yeah, I am on the weigh down again. Now I would like to dip below 150 to start the New Year. I want to start out the New Year in the 140s. That sounds like a reasonable goal for now to lose three pounds in the next six weeks. That is the goal I have for now. Tune in again tomorrow.

Be swift to exercise, slow to eat.

Ephesians 6:12

*For we wrestle not against flesh and blood, but against principalities, against powers, against the rulers of the darkness of this world, against spiritual wickedness in high places.*

For I wrestle not against flesh and food, but against food giants, marketing boards, lobbying boards, billboards, against the rulers of the darkness of fast food, against spiritual wickedness in the food industry.

November 23, 2011

I am not going to weigh myself again this year. I am annoyed that my weight today was up two pounds from last week and I can see no reason to have gained this week. It is too annoying and the first thing I wanted to do after getting on the scale was to eat. I didn't because I had to get off to work early. It is so defeating to have a gain and I struggle to convince myself to continue eating clean and working out when my weight doesn't drop. I could convince myself that the gain is muscle from weight lifting and that will suffice for today.

I remind myself that where the affections of my heart lie is reflected somewhat in the distribution and composition of fat in my body. What I truly love does show somewhat in what I have worshipped all the days of my life, whether that be food or God. When I get to the end of that straight and narrow path which leadeth to life eternal will I be narrow enough to fit through the gate and pass the Keeper of the gate who cannot be deceived by strategically placed scarves and slimming lines and basic black. Will He see where the affections of my heart have focused in the state of the body He created and gave to me? Will I be fit for the kingdom or too flabby to make the cut?

Have I finished my forty years in the wilderness?

# I have a dream

November 28, 2011

I have a dream that one day I will be able to sit down to a table of sumptuous food and not overeat. I have a dream that one day the daughters of food slaves and the daughters of the eternally fit will walk together united in love and sisterhood.

I have a dream that one day the state of my body will not be sweltering with the excess of fat and food, not sweltering with the injustice of food addiction, not sweltering from oversized thighs rubbing together, that one day it will be free of the oppression of food and fat.

I have a dream that one day my four beautiful children will live in a nation where they are not judged by the size of their thighs or their breasts or deltoids or gluts, but on the content of their character and measure of their love for others.

I have a dream that one day down in Hollywood, with its vicious fat-phobics that right there in that substation to hell, big fat men and big fat women will be able to walk hand in hand with big thin men and big thin women as brothers and sisters.

I have a dream that one day every fat cell shall be subdued, every lump and bulge and cellulite haven in my thighs shall be made smooth and my flesh shall be glorified in the Lord who created it.

I have a dream that one day the mountain of misery and discord on my thighs will be hewn down and replaced with the everlasting peace of God, and the jangling discords of my diet and food addicted soul will be replaced with the transformation to peace and joy in my body and soul.

I have a dream that one day I will be free from that awful monster, my food and diet obsession.

# Old diets die hard

December 14, 2011

I am reading in Mosiah chapter 1(*Book of Mormon*).

Without daily scripture study anyone could dwindle in unbelief. Without focusing on spiritual things daily my health resolves would dwindle as well. I can feel the gradual eroding of my determination to eat clean and healthy through the remainder of the year. I feel the old thinking creeping back into my mind and telling me to relax and eat what I want and take care of the consequences in January. Old habits die hard and bury themselves in my belly and thighs. I remind myself that over indulging will not bring peace or joy during the season. I need to rely on God to fight this battle for me and remember that sugar and treats and tarts and pies and shortbread are not love or joy or merriment. Rather they are misery and I do not want misery in my life. I want love, joy, peace, health, fitness and happy thighs. I guess without inspiring literature, I too am dwindling in my belief that food is not happiness and love and joy. I can celebrate without excess food. I need to remember the awful state I get into when I am using my drug of choice and how it leads to misery and anguish and shame and guilt and big thighs and butt and multiple chins and self-hatred. It's not worth the momentary pleasure of treats. The pleasure passes quickly while the misery of appetite continues as a flame of unquenchable craving that ascends up seemingly forever and it's not a fire that burns fat. It's a fire that ignites appetite—more and more and more and more. It's not a pretty picture.

I must consider the happy state I am in when I follow clean eating and eating in response to hunger rather than external cues all around me. Feeding my body should also feed my soul.

[Late evening] Ugh. Something went flatulently wrong between this morning and this evening. It all started when I decided to make treats to take to some friends. I found a recipe for Rice Krispy squares for the one with little kids then some peanut butter chocolate squares for the others. Off to the store I went to get the ingredients. Dumb idea! I should have given them poinsettias or something else not edible. As soon as I opened that can of sweetened condensed milk, I was stuck—lick, line, and sinker. I took a lick off the lid and that was the end of eating clean today. Ugh. I sampled everything several times and continued to eat them until I took them and gave them away. They are gone now and hopefully this is just a slip that will not carry on for the rest of the year. I have such a belly ache and flatulence like I haven't had all year, I swear. This is misery for sure and I am hoping that I don't end up with a migraine too. Next time I am tempted to make a treat I hope I change my mind and decide to be nice in some other way, non-edible way. Besides that I made a big mess in my kitchen and had to clean that up. It all makes no sense really. Now I am suffering with a terrible gut ache. I wish I could clean out that fat and sugar out of my digestive system as fast as I cleaned up the kitchen mess.

# Sugar happens

December 15, 2011

To continue the theme of last night, this is a situation where less is more for sure. Less of me physically means more abundance of joy and peace and hope and calm and all those things that go with spiritual and emotional health. I am grateful this morning that the firestorm in my gut has passed and I am feeling empty of the misery from yesterday's sugar binge except for a residual headache. It seems that for now all is calm in my colon and the tsunami of sugar gas has passed. Note to self again: Sugar is the substation to hell. How many memos and notes and emails and snail mails and FedEx's will it take for me to get the message internalized in my brain and belly and butt and thighs? I can call yesterday a slip, not a relapse, for my desire to conquer is still intact and I want today to be free from compulsive overeating.

This morning I am reading in Mosiah chapter 3 verse 18 (*Book of Mormon*), which talks about drinking damnation to my soul. I literally ate damnation to my soul yesterday. I felt the misery of the damned in the turmoil in my belly. If that isn't the torment of a damned colon I don't know what is! I suffered greatly at choir practice last night and was most grateful that I was removed enough from others in my pianist role that no one hopefully could hear or smell the torment going on in my gut. It was bad. It was lethal. And most stinky too.

The result of my sugar excess was that I was sitting in a smelly vapor agonizing over my rumbling gut while trying to play the piano for the Christmas choir. It was not a pretty or pleasantly aromatic picture. I was definitely fighting a firestorm of flatulence hell and my bowels were anything but filled with charity and love. They were filled with churning and burning and the smelly flatulence of the gluttonous damned. That is NOT a happy place to be. I would hate to have that be my eternal place of rest which would be anything but rest. That would be a situation of literally eating damnation to my soul.

Each day is judgement day when I am consigned to an awful or not awful view of my belly and butt, which may or may not cause me to shrink and hide out from others and myself. Each day is a judgement day of sorts when I judge what my final outcome will be, consigned to fat food hell or clean eating heaven.

Oh, remember my soul to no longer droop in sugar. Give place no more for the enemy of my soul and skinny jeans.

# Nothing new under the cellulite

<u>December 20, 2011</u>

There is nothing new under the sun, so the preacher in Ecclesiastes says. I suppose my cycle of journaling on weight and food issues rather supports the preacher's assertion. There has been nothing new under my dieting sun, only a cycle of the same thing over and over and over again. Yesterday I had a rather stressful day in ER and as the day progressed and my stress increased along with my hunger, I fell prey to the caramel popcorn, the muffins, and snacks sitting around. I noted no veggies sitting nearby and reminded myself that I could have been better prepared to face the onslaught of food along with the onslaught of the sick needing attention. I felt bad that I was feeling impatient with some and irritated at their demands so I ate to assuage my discomfort with the less than charitable feelings and that didn't help. It just made me more self-loathing.

I believe that my food rampages are somewhat fuelled by a desire to destroy myself or some part of myself. Perhaps when I see that which is good in me, I will have no desire to destroy myself. It's okay for me to be on the planet with both strengths and weaknesses.

That is how everyone else is. I am working to overcome my weaknesses as I develop my strengths. As I work towards developing my strengths, I am hopefully not taking up more than my share of air and space on the planet. I could say that literally as well as figuratively. I really don't want to take up more than my share of space here; I just want to be the size I am meant to be.

In church this past Sunday the lesson was on the final judgement in the *Gospel Principles* manual. It states that our bodies and minds will also be part of our judgement. "Stored in our body and mind is a complete history of everything we have done." I am writing a history of my life, not only in these lines, but also in the lines of my heart and my cellulite and my brain and my belly and chins and everywhere else. What a history my body must be writing over and over and over again with all its sizes and shapes and varying states of fitness and flabbiness. With each bite I eat and each workout I do I am writing my history and preparing my own final judgement. Yikes! So maybe after all the jokes and quips about being weighed and measured on judgement day, I actually WILL be weighed and measured on judgement day. My body really will be my autobiography written as I eat and walk and speak and think and write and run and dance and so forth.

It is now 8:00 p.m. and I am much too full. It started with chocolates at work then caramel popcorn then more chocolates and then real food in between then coming home and eating some chips (multigrain). I am totally off clean eating today and hoping to do better tomorrow and for the rest of this evening.

December 25, 2011

This is my last day of allowing excess food and I get back onto a clean eating schedule tomorrow.

December 26, 2011

I could pretend I didn't write that last entry and just delete it but my soul needs some integrity today. Some days I just want to eat and be a slug. I have worked a crazy busy shift at the hospital and the busier I got the more I ate—chocolates, cookies, squares, popcorn, candy, etc. Now my sugar-marinated brain is screaming for more and I just want to be a slug—no rules, no restraints, no resolutions, no plans, no goals, no sense. I just want to eat. The sluggish monster inside of me wants to express itself with endless, no calories barred food and that's what it's doing.

December 28, 2011

*Stand fast therefore in the liberty wherewith Christ hath made us free and be not entangled again with the yoke of bondage.* Galatians 5:1. I am sure that I have previously quoted this scripture but it seems fitting again today seeing that I am once again entangled in the yoke of sugar.

December 29, 2011

The psalmist speaks of those who have a double heart. I feel like I have a double heart. I am praying that the desire for sugar will leave me and yet I am romancing that peppermint ice-cream that is in my freezer left over from my family get together last night. More food and family and feasting. It just seems to go hand in hand, or more aptly, hand to mouth. Ah well, I can't live in a monastery, which is what seems to be what I need to do to avoid overeating. I guess that's how I kind of live when I am alone. I have much more control over my eating then.

December 31, 2011 3:30 a.m.

This Psalm 141 speaks to me this morning as I am suffering the insomnia of the damned or of the binged. *Set a watch, O Lord, before my mouth; keep the door of my lips.*

I feel good that I am smaller this year than last—about thirty pounds less. I'm not sure exactly how much because I haven't weighed myself for about a month and don't want to right now. I feel good about my fitness level.

Then 2011 turned into 2012 and I continued the eternal round of being me in varying sizes and shapes.

# Ruth's Proverb

January 13, 2012

Who can find a dieting woman for her price is far above calories?

The heart of her husband hath strayed far from her; she doth not trust in him. In dieting she trusts.

She won't be fat all the days of her life.

She seeketh squats and lunges, and worketh sweatingly with her hands, and legs, and gluts, and deltoids.

She is like the merchants' ships; she bringeth her fat free food from afar.

She ariseth also while it is yet night, and sweateth it up to the oldies and riles her buddies to sweat with her.

She considereth an exercise plan and buyeth it. With the strength of her hands she planteth her feet firmly into her Nike cross trainers and stompeth the ground wherein she walks.

She girdeth her thighs with strength and strengtheneth her arms.

She perceiveth that her fitness plan is good: her metabolism fire goeth not out by night.

She layeth her hands to the free weights and her feet to karate kicks.

She stretcheth out her hand to the fat; yea, she reacheth forth her hands to the obese.

She is not afraid of the snow for her walking, for all her body is clothed with scarves and mitts and toques and boots and silk leggings and snow joggers.

She maketh herself coverings of merino wool; her clothing is silk and purple.

Her husband is known no more for leaving her in the lurch, while he sitteth among the female haters of the land.

She buyeth spanx to cover her fat and squeeze her butt and thighs into coveted sizes. She covets her neighbor's ass, a firm size six.

Strength and sweat are her clothing and she shall rejoice in time to come.

She openeth her mouth less frequently and with calorie wise wisdom and in her tongue is the diet police.

She looketh well to the ways of her thighs and eateth not the bread of fatness.

Her children rise up and call her slim. Her husband left her long ago and doesn't give a nanocalorie.

Many daughters have dieted virtuously but thou excellest them all.

Favor is deceitful and beauty is vain, but a woman that escheweth fat, she shall be praised.

Give her of the fruit of her hands and let her own size praise her in the gates and halls and streets and forests.

# In and out and up and down

January 22, 2012

I faced the scale this morning for the first time in about two months and weighed 155 pounds. It's not bad considering my Christmas binge and all and then living off food storage this past month and not really eating clean, more like cleaning up the food in the house.

January 23, 2012

I love Deuteronomy 6: 4-10. I need to write the word 'remember' on my gate posts, walls, car window, wrist, neck, ankle, hands, fridge, garage, and mirrors to keep me in remembrance of the misery of compulsive overeating. I would rather have remembrance bound upon my neck than fat fastened to my thighs.

January 25, 2012 6:30 a.m.

I am reading in Alma 28 (*Book of Mormon*) and paraphrasing to liken it to me. The fat of many thousands of diets have I laid low in the earth while the fat of many thousands of binges is moldering in heaps upon my thighs. Hell would be a state of never ending dieting for sure, a state of endless weight. How great is the inequality of women because of metabolic rates and weights and size and the power of food.

Proverbs 11: 1. *A false balance is abomination to the Lord: but a just weight is his delight.*

Much of my life I have wanted the false balance. I have expected a weight that I wanted while eating that which gave me a just weight. I wanted the scale to say one thing while I stuffed myself with that which was contrary to the weight I wanted. Give me a just weight and give me the desire to eat according to the balance that I want.

It just dawned on me that if the world comes to an end this year as some have predicted (Mayan calendar) I certainly don't want to end up fat. I could call this my end of the world diet to get in shape for the final Armageddon. For me that will be the final and defining battle between fat and thin. Oh, oh, I have only eleven months now to win the battle. Will the threat of Armageddon be the ultimate impetus to propel me to that world of eternal slender?

I have been listening to *Remember When* by Alan Jackson. I could sing: remember when 130 pounds seemed so fat. Now, looking back, its right where I'd like to be.

February 2, 2012

Its groundhog's day today and I am thinking how much my life with diets reads like the movie *Groundhog's Day*. I just haven't seemed to be able to get out of it. Maybe I keep seeing my fat shadow and am frightened back into dieting obsessively until I am just a shadow of what I am, which hasn't yet happened.

Last night and tonight on the news there was a story about researchers in the US who are advocating that sugar is a toxic substance and should be taxed like alcohol and tobacco. I agree. I know from my experience that it is very toxic to me. Here is a direct quote from the article on sugar tax: '*Sugar is as damaging and addictive as alcohol or tobacco and should be regulated, claim US health experts.*' I agree with this. I have never drank or smoked but I have certainly been tormented with sugar and I can only imagine the torment of other addictions being very similar to mine.

# The mother of all diets

February 25, 2012

I was thinking about John's [Revelations] visions of the final roundup of the last days. My own vision would be like this:

I saw the mother of all diets arrayed in stripes and black colors and a scarf of pure spun sugar was draped around her neck to draw all eyes to her face and not her thighs. She was decked with long golden onion rings and bracelets of pretzels and a ring of chocolate in her nose. In her hands she carried a golden cup filled with protein shakes and Slimfast shakes and elderberry fasts and HCG and Atkins bars and she wielded them with the determination of the dieting damned. Her mouth was filled with blasphemous diets and she had seven chins and four breasts filled with the fat of the dieting damned. Upon her forehead was emblazoned, mystery of misery, "the great mother of all diets and mistress of misery to the women of the earth." I saw the woman drunken with the cellulite of the saints and crying dieting to all. When I saw her I trembled with great fear and my cellulite jiggled and I sought deep to hide my thighs and chins and belly flab.

I watched her fat fall and great was the fall thereof, sinking deeper and deeper into the bottomless pit of dieting, drowning in her Slimfast shakes and elderberry fasts, and HCG, the pit from whence no sanity can come and I struggled against her magnetic pull sucking me into another diet fad, but in the end I let her go. She is not joy. She is not peace. She is not that promised land of eternal slender that I seek. She is only the evils and designs of a conspiring diet industry in the last days, bent on destroying the peace and pocketbooks of unsuspecting women who just want to be loved and thin.

# Still hungry after all these years

March 15, 2012

I don't even know why I stepped on the scale this morning. I guess because I felt slim but my mood shot down again by a flipping number on the scale. Now I am just mad again about my weight. I weigh 159 pounds and I am bemused, befuddled, and befatted. Why am I 159 pounds? I work out, do weights, walk, wish, and pine and pray and eat what I consider to be moderate. Okay, okay, I am sounding like stuff fat women say now. I don't eat that much! My denying brain tricks may be once again forefront and I am really not admitting to what and how much I eat. I really don't want to be in a downer mood all day because of a stupid number on the scale. So awake my soul, no longer droop in size. What do I lack yet? It must be time to start again recording everything that goes into my mouth. I hear that is a strategy of those who have long time weight loss success. Waist management is getting to be very time consuming and tedious. It's becoming a 24/7 job like parenting. Maybe that is what I need—a parent again to manage me. Or I need a lady in weighting or a food nanny just to manage my weight and nothing else. Wait a minute, that hasn't seemed to help notorious celebrities who struggle up and down with their weight issues, so how could it help a struggling peasant like me? Still hungry after all these years.

Not there yet, wherever there is.

# The bucket of food list

A friend asked me one day if I had a bucket list of things I wanted to do before I die. I don't but I have had several buckets of food lists mentally itemizing everything Iwanted to eat before I diet. I have had many D days, the dreaded day when a diet was to start so in the days leading up to that D day I stuffed myself every waking minute in an attempt to eat everything I might be missing and more by going on the dreaded diet. These bucket lists have included pizza (chicken club with extra cheese), nachos and cheese (not the low fat kind), breadsticks with extra cheese, ice-cream, ice-cream, ice- cream, cheesecake, smokies with cheese, and throw in a few of my favorite candy bars *Eatmore* (that should tell me something!). In fact, I ate stuff that I never would have eaten anyway if I hadn't been planning an infernal diet. Go figure! More like GONE figure. I notice that this list does not include any vegetables or fruit or cottage cheese or flax which is a shame because I actually do like these foods until I get into the go-on-a-diet mentality and then I eat all the crap I think I might miss. I know. It doesn't make any sense but neither does the government or weather or my dieting history really.

# Much dieting hath made me mad

I am mad that so much of my life energy has been consumed with dieting. I am mad that even with all that, I am still tempted by every wind of diet that blows my way. I am most mad that despite all this I am not slim. I am mad that I haven't yet conquered the enemy of my soul. I am mad that so much of my life enjoyment I have put on hold until that magic day when I would be slim. I am so mad that I have to work so hard just to not gain weight.

In all this madness, what have I learned in over forty years of dieting? Seemingly not a damn thing because I continue to struggle as I write this now and wonder if this will be my thorn in the cellulite until I die. And maybe even after that when I could be consigned forever to food hell, not necessarily a hot place but a fat place. Maybe hell for me would be sentenced to life forever around the perennially thin who can't understand why I would continue to eat when I am full, or continue to eat until I vomit then eat some more, then be mad when I want to continue to eat but there is no room left in my stomach or colon or esophagus, not even room left in my oral cavity or sinuses or aural cavities.

Yes, that would be an even greater hell than fat hell, to dwell with the eternally thin who have no understanding of the power of food over me. I know they would be eternally judging me for my inability to get my cellulite together. Better to live with the damned fat souls in hell than to be eternally racked with torment by being surrounded by the thin!

I don't hate thin people, don't get me wrong. I just envy them with every fiber of my cellulite and I wish I could be one of them instead of two of them like I am.

But then again, if I were a perennially thin person I may have missed discovering the joy of walking and the joy of weights and the joy of losing weight over and over and over again. That's a whole lot of joy to be missing out on in one life time. If I were always thin I would not have had the motivation to exercise and sweat and grunt and cycle and so forth. I may also have missed the health benefits of eating nutritious food in my quest for thinness.

My fat has been my principal motivator for exercise and for eating nutritiously and has brought me so much joy in that sick kind of roundabout way that adversity brings joy, if that's what I can call this thorn in the flesh that I have. I would also not have been motivated to learn about twelve-step work and all the lessons I have learned through seeking a solution to my weight obsession. There you have it, right there in thick and thin: fat has been a blessing in my life and will likely continue to be as I crawl the walk of recovery.

# The school of fat knocks

I guess I have learned a thing or two (random things really) from my numerous attempts to be slim. I have learned that death by chocolate really is death by chocolate (think migraines that make you wish your head was cut off).

I have learned not to bask in weight loss. It doesn't stick. It's kind of like the stock market with ups and downs and little predictability. I am weary with having a variable weight. I want a fixed weight for a change, fixed between 130 and 135 pounds. That would give me a five-pound variability up or down and yet stay that magic size of my dreams.

I have learned that it's never over, even after the fat lady slims down **and** sings.

I have learned that being thin feels better than being fat, and yet, I rarely stay slim when I get there. I have learned that I seem to be treated differently depending on my size. When I am slim I seem to get more positive attention and respect. But maybe that is just my perception because I treat myself differently when I am slim and I dress myself with greater care. I have more respect for myself and perhaps that gives me the illusion that others have more respect for me as well.

I have learned that no amount of money can buy slimness, just as no amount of money can buy heaven or happiness or love or laughter. I can't seem to buy my way into a size and stay there. Not that I have had tons of money but I have spent a considerable amount on diet books and diet foods and diet programs and exercise programs and the ever changing sizes of clothing in my closet. No amount of money seems to compensate for whatever is missing in my soul.

I have learned that my memory is very much clouded, likely with sugar, when it comes to remembering how much I have eaten and the subsequent head pain and peristaltic pain and heart pain of binging over and over and over again. Why else would I repeat this fattening and flatulent routine over and over and over again?

I have learned that no matter how much I imagine and visualize and wish and chant and ponder and pray, I cannot defy the universal laws of nature. The excess food I eat DOES land somewhere in my body whether I tell it otherwise or not. Despite visualizing and chanting that no matter what I eat I can stay size six and no matter how much I command those calories to exit my body, they do not go. They land on my thighs because I ate too much. I have learned that I can choose what I eat but I cannot choose the consequences of what I eat. I cannot chant or visualize or wish or pray away the laws of nature.

I have learned that I am not a dress size. I am SEVERAL dress sizes. From size eight to size sixteen, I keep my closet packed and ready for any relapse or binge or diet.

I have learned that many of my dieting attempts have just been scratch the surface solutions, just like scratch the surface housekeeping where I only got through the first layer but never went beyond to clean up and clear out what was really eating me up. I need to go much deeper into my soul and at the same time much higher into the realms of God to beat the demons that I have fed and coddled and catered to all these years. This is not so much a destination as it is a never ending journey.

I have learned that I don't go away no matter what I weigh or where I live, I stay me. I have fought this fat fight in the Canadian provinces of British Columbia, Ontario, Quebec, and Alberta. I have fought it in Utah. I have fought it in Hong Kong, Thailand, and the islands of the Philippines. I have fought it on the beaches of Hawaii, Mexico, and Cuba. I have fought it in India and in flights over the ocean. In all these places I have been me or rather, variable versions of me.

I have learned that everyone has their own god of sorts that they choose to worship. This god may be food, or drink, or diet, or self, or money, or power, or hockey or whatever else we mortals may carry around for decades until willingness to let them go brings us to the point that we do let go.

I have learned that I will never be enough and that's okay. I don't have to be. I have God to pick up the slack where I cannot.

I have learned that no matter how strong I feel and no matter how much I think that I have conquered my weakness, it returns again and again both when I least expect it and when I most expect it too. Arrival is not an option. I have learned that until I am immortal, I am mortal. It's simple really and as a mortal perhaps this is my cross to bear or more aptly put my cellulite to bear.

I have watched my diet crazed journey span a number of developmental phases from adolescence to adulthood, or so I thought, but maybe I never really left adolescence. Perhaps I have been continually trying to resolve my adolescent identity over and over and over again ad nauseam, not so much trying to find myself as trying to hide myself.

I am learning just for today that it's finally okay for me to be me, to come out of the pantry and quit hiding in the pretzels and pizza and potatoes.

Then again, if I was trying to hide then making myself bigger was certainly not a very effective way to hide. Perhaps in a twisted bloated sense of puffed up self, maybe I really was trying to be found rather than trying to hide.

In all this learning I have journeyed to the innermost depths of my heart and colon and seen and written what I have found there—the thin, the fat, and the ugly. I am purging it out one moment, one calorie, one prayer, one walk at a time. In this journey of searching and fearless purging I have found what was missing most in my life (Surprise! It wasn't a man). It was me! The real me, the divine me, the me that God intended to be me.

Now I bid farewell until we all shall meet chin to chin and thigh to thigh before that great and dreadful judgement scale in the sky where all will be weighed and measured and scanned and scrutinized. In all this judging and weighing and measuring and scanning may we all be found fit for a kingdom in God's house of many sizes.

# About the Author

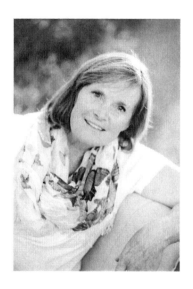

Ruth was born and raised in the back woods of British Columbia. In addition to a nursing degree she has a PhD in psychology. Her passion for writing has filled many notebooks and journals from mid teens to midlife. She lives in the beautiful Creston Valley with her piano, her scale, and her diets.

CPSIA information can be obtained at www.ICGtesting.com
Printed in the USA
LVOW060954180113

316172LV00001B/21/P